$4⁹⁵

NATURAL HORMONES
The Secret of Youthful Health

Other Books by the Author:

Helping Your Health with Enzymes

Magic Minerals: Key to Better Health

The Natural Way to Health Through Controlled Fasting

Carlson Wade's Gourmet Health Foods Cook Book

Natural and Folk Remedies

The Natural Laws of Healthful Living

Health Tonics, Elixirs and Potions for the Look and Feel of Youth

NATURAL HORMONES
The Secret of Youthful Health

Carlson Wade

Parker Publishing Company, Inc.　　　　West Nyack, N.Y.

Printed in the United States of America
ISBN 0-13-609941-6
B & P

DEDICATION

To Your Renewed
Youthful Health

FOREWORD

By a Doctor of Medicine

Nature has placed a set of "biological clocks" within the human body that serve as the source of healthfully timed, youthful vigor at all ages. In the form of glands, these nature-created "clocks" are properly adjusted by corrective hormone food programs, "live" fruit, vegetable and seed juices, simple exercises, home water therapy, and other wholesome methods. These all-natural programs are known to help adjust and alert the glandular clocks, to enable them to issue forth a properly timed "hormone rhythm" which is basically the secret of youthful health.

In this carefully researched and commendable book, there is a remarkable collection of all-natural "gland rejuvenation" programs, the use of simple nature plants and foods for "hormone enrichment," and enjoyable, yet remarkably effective, time-tested corrective eating and living programs. All help your glands pour forth youth-building hormones to build and rebuild body-mind health.

This unique book calls for restoration of nature's healthy hormones with tasty foods, delicious tonics, and enjoyable home programs. They benefit the glands by helping to alert and adjust them to precision-timing hormone rhythm and boosting a feeling of youth from the inside to the outside.

It is encouraging to see that the simple programs call for all-natural ingredients, speedily prepared, helping to put nature into your glands and youth into your hormones.

Carlson Wade's new book is highly recommended to those who want to use nature to help improve their health and enjoy the youth-building benefits of natural hormones.

Leslie H. Salov, M.D

What This Book Can Do for You

Throughout my career as a health reporter and writer of many health books and articles, I have hopefully researched the "secrets" of youthful health. Many of the authorities consulted told about "miraculous rejuvenation" made possible through a regenerated supply of natural hormones. Furthermore, persons could experience the look and feel of youth when particular programs and folk remedies using *Hormone Foods*—certain common foods that help stimulate your hormone-producing glands—were used.

These authorities described many case histories. They offered step-by-step, all-natural programs—using Hormone Foods— in which the body's glands could be healthfully adjusted and recharged to issue the vital hormones that held the key to prolonged youth of body and mind.

Success after success was reported. Hormones from natural sources helped put a youthful glow into people in all walks of life, of all ages, under different circumstances. These reported case histories told how natural hormones gave much more than just the appearance of youth. The overall benefit was a joy of youthful health in meeting the challenges of daily living, thanks to natural hormones.

This book is a treasury of these "secret hormone food methods." They were previously known to only a select few who reaped the rewards of renewed youthful looks and a "forever young" feeling through natural hormones. Now, you are able to share in these secrets. You can now help give your body the supply of youth-building hormones it may need, to give yourself the look and feel of healthy youthfulness—at any age!

This book shows you how to use these secrets of nature, to help stimulate youthful hormone production of your endocrine glands. It gives you lists of special foods, special folk remedies from all parts of the world, and easy-to-follow natural programs. It shows you how to use nature's own "hormone foods" to give you the zest of life, the spirit of youthful health.

9

When you follow these programs, you help create hormone harmony within your body, the foundation of youthful health. Once you build this hormone foundation, you are then able to help your body and mind experience the benefits of rejuvenation. Soon you can begin to look and feel younger. This book furnishes you this guidance. The step-by-step programs, taken from documented reports, help you achieve your goal of youthfulness through hormones from natural sources.

Every chapter in this book is programmed to offer you an easy, step-by-step method you can follow—completely illustrated with reported case histories of those who awakened their glands and reaped the rewards of youthfulness through natural hormone foods. Every chapter is a rich source of this knowledge, as drawn from worldwide research that spans several centuries—right up to our present space age—to help you claim the youthfulness you desire.

Many names have been used to describe this method in these pages. However, each one is descriptive of the same method—*Natural Hormones: The Secret of Youthful Health.*

All remedies and step-by-step programs in this book are medicine-less. They are all-natural—no expensive drugs of any kind required. All listed ingredients are available for pennies without prescription in your local supermarket, health foods store, or herbalist. You probably have many of these items presently in your refrigerator or cupboard.

It is surprisingly simple to follow this method. It is a most satisfying experience to enjoy the benefits of a healthy hormone system as programmed for you in this book—the secret of looking and feeling younger with dynamic health.

Carlson Wade

Table of Contents

NATURAL HORMONES
The Secret of Youthful Health

1

The Secret of Restoring and Keeping Youthfulness with Natural Hormones

You are as youthful as the health of your glandular system! You are as energetic as the health of your glands! You are as mentally alert as the health of your glands! Within your body and mind, you have a set of seven nature-created "fountains" which issue forth "gushing springs" of body-mind substances that help put youthful life into nearly all of your voluntary and reflex processes. These "fountains" are your basic endocrine glands. These "gushing springs" are your glandular secretions of hormones—the secret of youthful health.

How Natural Health Programs Set Your Biological Gland Clocks

By following all-natural health programs, you can help set up your internal "biological gland clocks" to function adequately by means of "hormone rhythm balance" to further promote a feeling of youthful health. Your seven nature-created endocrine glands need "adjustment" by means of proper nutrition and time-tested exercises, as well as corrective hormone food programs. Once your "biological gland clocks" have been "adjusted" by natural health programs, they are able to "tick" smoothly by issuing a healthful supply of youth-building hormones—the very key to your life and health.

An 11-Point Natural Hormone Food Program to "Wind Up" Your "Biological Gland Clocks"

Your body should be a healthy "hormone fountain" that is rhythmically "in tune" with your "biological gland clocks." Given the proper and all-natural "windup" with healthful hormone foods and natural living programs, the clocks should tick forth a smooth and rhythmic movement of these youth-giving hormones. Recognizing that much ill health may well be traced to a "slowed up" gland clock, a physician treated over 700 patients by "winding up" their endocrine gland network until the "hormone fountains" ticked away in a rhythmic flow of youth-bestowing benefits. The doctor was able to promote healing amongst these patients by suggesting an 11-point program that reportedly helped correct hormonal imbalances. The doctor[1] found that natural nutrition and hormone foods could well adjust a malfunctioning "biological gland clock" and promote a look and feel of youth for body and mind. Here is the 11-Point Natural Program that helps adjust the endocrine gland network to a more healthful rhythm:

1. Serve as many hormone foods in the natural state as possible. These include raw, fresh fruits and vegetables, certified whole milk, fresh butter, natural and non-processed cheeses, and cold-pressed vegetable oils. *GLANDULAR BENEFITS:* Raw and non-processed hormone foods are prime sources of enzymes that are needed to stimulate the body's network of endocrine glands. These raw food enzymes act as "energizers" or "spark plugs" to the body's glands and help them initiate manufacture of their gushing hormones.

2. Your hormone food program should emphasize a high protein content. Good sources include the variety meats (liver, brain, heart), poultry, and sea food. Include dairy products: eggs, non-processed cheese, and certified milk. *GLANDULAR BENEFITS:* The body's glands need protein to nourish the cells and tissues, as well as the intricate arterial tubules and valves with which they are interconnected. Protein helps furnish the "power" used by glands to issue forth their supply of youth-giving hormones.

3. Use fresh fruits and vegetables (grown without the use of poisonous chemical sprays, wherever possible). Cook vegetables with

---

[1]J.D. Walters, M.D., *Journal of Applied Nutrition,* Vol. 10, Winter Issue.

a minimum of water, and for as short a time as possible. Drink the water in which the vegetables were cooked. *GLANDULAR BENE-FITS:* Fresh or slightly cooked foods are prime sources of vitamins and minerals which help to regulate body water balance and enter into the manufacture of hormones; *the hormones, themselves, are partially made of vitamins and minerals, which must come from fresh and wholesome fruits and vegetables.* To have "rich hormones," feed your glands an abundance of these fresh foods.

4. Use freshly ground whole-grain cereals and flours. These are good sources of protein, the valuable B-complex vitamins, precious Vitamin E, as well as unsaturated fatty acids. *GLANDULAR BENE-FITS:* These nutrients help "wind up" and also "oil" the "gland clocks" and enable them to tick forth a steady and soothing supply of hormone rhythm. Without the "oil" from these natural foods, the "machinery" of the "gland clocks" may become sluggish and malfunctioning.

5. Use cold-pressed vegetable or seed oils as an excellent source of essential unsaturated fatty acids. *GLANDULAR BENEFITS:* The "gland clocks" are subject to accumulations of "sludge" or cholesterol deposits caused by an excessive intake of hard fats which surround the meat or are "marbled" into it. The use of unsaturated and cold-pressed seed oils will help "clean" the "rust" from the body's network of "gland clocks" and promote a smooth and well-oiled, efficient bodily mechanism.

6. Eliminate the use of refined sugar in all forms. Substitute natural sweets, such as honey (in moderation) or rose hips powder, carob powder, date powder, blackstrap molasses. *GLANDULAR BENEFITS:* Refined sugar creates an acid condition in the system and will tend to leave a harsh "residue" upon the "gland clocks," impeding their healthful function. An excessive amount of refined sugar also speeds up the body metabolism as it seeks to process the unnatural amount of sweets; this calls for overwork by the body's glands and there may follow internal exhaustion. Use natural and wholesome sweets, in moderation.

7. Eliminate the use of bleached white flour products. The valuable nutrients of the whole grain have been removed. Frequent bleaching and preservative agents are added and create disharmony amongst the body's gland networks. *GLANDULAR BENEFITS:* Bleached white flour products cause a harsh and volatile reaction upon the endocrine glands; the chemicals in artificially preserved flour products further impede natural glandular function and may cause unrest and ill health.

8. Eliminate the use of foods which contain chemical additives—these include packaged bread, pastries, ice cream, and cold or prepared-cured meats. These are saturated with preservatives, artificial coloring and chemical flavoring agents, synthetic emulsifiers, extenders, sweeteners, stabilizers, etc. *GLANDULAR BENEFITS:* The glands of your body must draw their substance from the food you eat. If you feed your glands an assortment of artificial chemicals, then the hormones they manufacture will have a high content of these toxic substances. Such "chemical-filled hormones" can cause disarray in your hormone rhythm. Instead, feed your glands a supply of wholesome and natural foods from which they can make healthful and youth-giving hormones.

9. Eliminate the use of poultry and meats produced with hormones to stimulate animal growth and add weight. *GLANDULAR BENEFITS:* These animal hormones that have been injected into the bird in the form of synthetic chemicals may find their way into your own hormone system. It is as gland-risky as mixing different qualities of gasoline in the tank of your automobile. The end result is an internal upheaval that may require the help of a costly and, perhaps, painful specialist. Instead, select wholesome and organic meats that have not been tainted by injections of chemical hormones.

10. Eliminate the use of hydrogenated (hard or saturated) fats and oils. They are excessively high in saturated fatty acids. Substitute with seed and vegetable oils. *GLANDULAR BENEFITS:* An excessive amount of "hard fats" may accumulate on the delicate cells and tissues of the glands and slow down their function; the "gland clock" may become overburdened with the heavy sludge and tick forth a reduced and less-than-perfect supply of hormones. This may lead to an overall decline in body functions. *Suggestion:* Use cold-pressed natural seed and vegetable oils to help lubricate your "gland clocks" so they can tick forth a supply of "hormone rhythm."

11. Eliminate excessive use of heated or processed milk, processed cheese, and processed cheese food spreads and products. *GLANDULAR BENEFITS:* These heated and processed dairy products have experienced a marked reduction in their perishable vitamins-minerals-enzymes. Furthermore, some of the proteins may also have been altered by the processing, and this creates an unfavorable reaction in your glandular network. Processed foods are treated with preservatives and artificial additives, which may find their way into the eventual hormones that come gushing throughout your body, splashing the delicate organs with their volatile power. Body function may decline when the hormones are excessively chemicalized.

How This All-Natural Hormone Food Program Promoted Youthful Healing Through Glandular Nourishment. The doctor was able to help his patients reset and readjust their "biological gland clocks" through the use of an all-natural hormone food program, as outlined above. Some of his patients suffered from allergies, arthritis, asthma, heart conditions, diabetes, ulcers, infertility, obesity, and skin disease. Others had chronic colds. *Nearly all displayed symptoms of premature aging—typical of malfunctioning of the glandular network.* By prescribing an all-natural hormone food program to help strengthen and rejuvenate the glands, the doctor was able to promote healing in almost all of the 700 patients. Once they had a healthful flow of youth-giving hormones, their health problems subsided and they were soon on the way to recovery. Thus we see the tremendous influence on health that is produced by the body's "gland clocks" and their "hormone rhythm."

Your Seven "Gland Clocks" and How to "Adjust" Them for Youthful Health

Locked within your body are seven basic "gland clocks" that need proper "adjustment" to help promote the look and feel of youthful health. By means of all-natural hormone food programs, you can help "adjust" these "clocks" to enable them to tick forth a steady supply of "hormone rhythm." Let's see how this can work to improve your body-mind feeling of health.

1. *The Pituitary Gland.* About the size of a pea, it hangs from a short stalk at the base of the brain. Though tiny, the pituitary is called the "master gland," because its three lobes secrete at least nine known hormones, and it regulates more complex body functions than are known for any other endocrine gland. *Pituitary Hormones Produce:* ACTH, (adreno-corticotropic-hormone) which stimulates the cortex of the adrenals to secrete its hormones; gonadotropin, which influences sexual development and production of sex hormones; prolactin, which promotes secretion of breast milk in the pregnant female; pancreatropin, which affects production of insulin; somatotropin, which regulates bone growth; thyrotropin, which regulates the thyroid gland; oxytocin, which stimulates uterine contractions and breast milk release; vasopressin, which affects blood pressure and water excretion.

How to Adjust Your Pituitary Gland Clock. This gland depends upon a sufficient supply of all the valuable nutrients, especially minerals. The gland "soaks up" minerals, which it then includes in its hormones to help regulate normal blood pressure, promote mental alertness, and maintain a youthful appearance, strong bones, and healthful nerve responses. You can adjust your Pituitary Gland Clock with these basic hormone food materials:

Morning Mineral Tonic. In a glass of tomato juice, squeeze the juice of one-half lemon. Add two tablespoons of celery juice, stir vigorously. Lastly, add one tablespoon of desiccated liver (a powdered form of liver from which the fat and connective tissues have been removed and a prime source of gland-feeding minerals). Stir again until all is assimilated as fluid. Drink in the morning. *Special Benefit:* The pituitary gland responses are slower in the morning after having been "turned down" for the night. Therefore, a Morning Mineral Tonic can spell all the difference between a youthful day and a tired day! Wind up your Pituitary Gland Clock in the morning with this healthful mineral tonic.

Brewer's Yeast Brain Food. Brewer's Yeast is regarded as a powerhouse of the B-complex vitamins that are needed by the nerve cells, which form a lacy network over the pea-sized Pituitary Gland Clock. When you mix two tablespoons of Brewer's Yeast (available in powdered form at specialty food shops or health stores) in a cup of non-processed or natural cottage cheese, you are stirring up a potent source of vitamins and essential minerals. In combination, these are taken up by the pituitary to be metabolized into healthful hormones that then "tick off" to promote a youthful alertness for most of the day.

Suggestions: Raw fresh fruits and vegetables, as well as their freshly squeezed juices, are prime sources of vitamins-minerals-enzymes that are needed by the pituitary gland as "food" to help it manufacture the vital hormones to keep your body-mind network in youthful function. Take frequent "juice breaks" throughout the day. Your Pituitary Gland Clock can thus be wound up frequently through all-natural, fresh, raw juices.

2. *The Thyroid Gland.* A two-part endocrine gland, it looks like a butterfly and rests against the front of the windpipe. *Thyroid Hormones Produced:* Both thyroxine and tri-iodothyronine work to regulate the rate of metabolism, the process by which hormone food is transferred into nutrients to be used by the body and mind to promote youthful health. Some people are thin, nervous, high-strung, and do everything rapidly with nervous gestures. Others are chubby,

slow-moving, and inclined to be lazy. One reason for these differences in health and personality may well be the difference in makeup and health of the thyroid gland.

How to Adjust Your Thyroid Gland Clock. There is one "magic mineral" hormone food that actually serves the prime purpose of "winding up" the thyroid gland so it can then issue forth its healthful hormones. That mineral is *iodine*—the mineral that energizes the gland to manufacture valuable thyroxine. Other vitamins and minerals as well as proteins and enzymes also help alert this gland, but *iodine* is the star of all and the "key" that unlocks a slow-moving Thyroid Gland Clock so it can move in harmonious rhythm and issue the valuable thyroxine hormone. Here's how to wind up your Thyroid Gland Clock:

Iodine Concentrate. At most pharmacies, health stores, special food shops, herbalists, you will be able to obtain one single tablet containing a daily iodine supply. To wind up your Thyroid Gland Clock, take just one tablet daily, with a glass of fresh vegetable juice. *Benefits:* The iodine is used by the thyroid to issue the valuable thyroxine hormone, which then works with amino acids (metabolized proteins) in the body to enter the bloodstream. Here, the iodine-rich thyroxine hormone works to build skin color, enrich the blood, firm up and rejuvenate muscles, stabilize weight, promote mental alertness, boost energy output, and help promote a healthful emotional temperament. Indeed, it is a miracle of hormone power—from a tiny iodine tablet!

Fresh Seafood. Because food iodine comes basically from the oceans, seafood is a good source of this valuable thyroid gland food. Obtain healthful seafood and try to eat it at least twice or three times weekly, for a good iodine as well as mineral source of thyroid gland food.

Hormone Youth Elixir. Kelp is a form of powdered seaweed which is regarded as a potent and naturally powerful source of iodine. It is a good source of essential minerals that become food for the thyroid. Make yourself an Hormone Youth Elixir by mixing one-half teaspoon of kelp powder (sold at most natural food outlets and herbalists, too) in a glass of fresh vegetable juice. Stir in one-half teaspoon of desiccated liver. Stir vigorously and then sip slowly. *Benefits:* The thyroid gland will collect the iodine from the kelp and several amino acids from the liver, combine them with the nutrients in the vegetable juice, and help make thyroxine, the hormone that determines youthful metabolism and a feeling of good health

How Mary T. Was Rejuvenated with Hormone Foods. At age 35, Mary T. was experiencing symptoms of premature aging. Her internal organs were improperly functioning, she developed a skin rash at the nape of her neck and the palm of one hand. She had emotional and physical difficulties that failed to respond to other forms of medication.

The doctor's treatment now consisted of winding up her thyroid gland. He did this by giving Mary T. this simple program:

1. *Iodine Supplement.* She was to take a daily supplement of an iodine food supplement capsule to help nourish her thyroid.

2. *Seed Oils.* Mary T. was to use cod liver oil, seed oils, and unheated salad oils on her fresh, raw salads—and also mix vegetable juices with them. This helped lubricate a "rusty" Thyroid Gland Clock.

3. *Starch Reduction and Vitamin-Mineral Boosting.* She was to reduce excess starch foods; she was also to take vitamin-mineral supplemental capsules. This helped stimulate her sluggish endocrine gland network and helped all the glands to work in harmonious rhythm.

Benefits: This all-natural program, which called for the use of the simple 11-Point Natural Hormone Food Program at the start of this chapter, helped adjust Mary T.'s biological "Thyroid Gland Clock." With a healthy stream of hormones, her premature aging symptoms subsided, her skin condition cleared up, and in three months, she was pronounced fit and healthy. Reportedly, an alerted thyroid gland had brought her back to the world of youthful living!

Suggestions: Freshly cooked seafood should be part of your twice-weekly food program. Iodine supplements are reportedly gland soothing. Follow the basic principles of natural nutrition to help wind up your thyroid and other glands.

3. *The Parathyroid Glands.* Each, about the size of a pea, are located at the four corners of the thyroid. *Parathyroid Hormone Produced:* Parathormone works to regulate the use of phosphorus and calcium by body tissues. Too little of this hormone may cause a condition of muscle spasms, cramps, and convulsions. Other distress signals may be erratic heartbeat, irritable nerves, loss of normal sight and hearing, and poor appetite. *Note:* Malnourished parathyroids may lead to kidney distress because of faulty calcium metabolism. The "key" to winding up the Parathyroid Glands Clock is found in

maintaining a healthful calcium-phosphorus balance. A slight alteration may cause maladjustment of body processes.

How to Adjust Your Parathyroid Glands Clock. Prime sources of nourishment will be found in hormone foods such as non-processed cheeses, soybean milk, and natural dairy products. Note that all the minerals in the world will do little good in the body, unless the parathyroid hormone is also present in the bloodstream to control and distribute these minerals. While controlling the body metabolism of calcium, the parathyroids, themselves, need calcium to keep "wound up" and to issue forth the valuable hormone that helps metabolize other body nutrients. Following are some all-natural suggestions:

Bone Meal Tonic. Bone meal powder—available at most health food shops and herbal pharmacies—together with soy milk, becomes a Bone Meal Tonic that is a most powerful source of gland-feeding calcium. If you will just mix two heaping tablespoons of bone meal powder in the soy milk and drink several glasses throughout the day, you will help feed your parathyroid gland.

Parathyroid Hormone Energizer. In one glass of milk, add one tablespoon of Brewer's Yeast. Stir vigorously and drink. *Benefit:* The natural supply of calcium and phosphorus in both the milk and the Brewer's Yeast form a balance of mineral food for the parathyroids. This is then used for energizing these glands and to help their glandular "clock" tick forth its valuable supply of parathormone, which is needed to maintain a healthful metabolic harmony in the body.

4. *The Thymus Gland.* This endocrine gland is located in the upper part of the chest, under the breastbone; specifically, it is situated on the windpipe below the thyroids. *Thymus Hormone Produced:* Retine is the hormone that is said to be involved with the body's immunity-building system; it also helps and assists in growth factors and usually ceases to function in young adulthood. But until this young adulthood is reached, the Thymus Gland Clock should be carefully adjusted to help promote healthy growth.

How to Adjust Your Thymus Gland Clock. Metabolism of minerals, especially *calcium* and *phosphorus,* is the chief known function of the thymus, and they are needed by this gland for its power. *NOTE:* A lack of the B-complex vitamins may cause impairment of mineral metabolization, and the thymus gland may become "wound down" because of this deficiency. To help wind up the Thymus Gland Clock, your food program should include ample minerals and also the B-complex vitamins. Here are tips on how to wind up your Thymus Gland Clock:

Homemade Mineral Milk. Use only non-pasteurized, certified raw milk. Place a bottle of this milk in a pan filled with tepid water. Now warm to about body temperature. Pour into four cups. Into each cup, stir one tablespoon of yogurt. Cover with a paper towel (to keep out dust) and put in a warm place (close to the stove or heating radiator, or wherever you have a consistent warm temperature). Let it remain there for 24 hours. Then eat this Homemade Mineral Milk with a spoon. This is an old-fashioned way of making yogurt or "soured milk," yet it is a powerhouse of valuable minerals needed by the thymus and other "biological gland clocks."

Oriental Gland Food. For hundreds of years, the Orientals have used a special "gland food" that appears to work miracles for the thymus, as well as other body glands. The secret here may be in the tremendous treasure of minerals, vitamins, enzymes, and, most important, the B-complex vitamins which work with calcium and phosphorus to help wind up the thymus clock so it can issue its valuable immunity-building hormones. Here's how to make this Oriental Gland Food:

    1 cup sesame seeds
    1/4 cup natural wheat germ flakes
    3 teaspoons dark honey

Grind sesame seeds in an electric seed grinder until a meal is formed. Pour into a larger cup. Next knead the honey into the meal, using a large spoon. When the honey is well mixed, add the wheat germ flakes. You continue kneading and mixing until it acquires the shape of a hard dough. You may serve in small balls or bars. It is something like halvah (Turkish candy). It is a treasure of gland food! A tasty confection from the Orient, where long and healthful lives are often the envy of the rest of the world.

5. *The Adrenal Glands Clock.* A pair of glands, shaped something like Brazil nuts, located astride each kidney, like that of a "cocked hat," are the adrenals. *Adrenal Glands Hormones Produced:* The *cortex* (covering) issues cortin, a hormone complex (including cortisone, hydrocortisone, and aldosterone) which controls the salt and water balance in the body; this hormone complex also influences the metabolization of carbohydrates, fat, and protein, maintains resistance to stress such as heat, cold, and poisons, influences muscular efficiency, and reduces inflammation and allergy. The *medulla* (central portion) issues adrenaline which rouses physical activity and

causes constriction of blood vessels, increased heart action, and nervous system arousal. *NOTE:* In times of danger or stress extra adrenaline is released into the bloodstream, where it works to increase the energy-yielding sugar in the blood, slows up or stops digestion, sluices blood into the big muscles, and dilates the pupils of the eyes; it may even cause the hair to stand on end. This hormone prepares the body to meet emergencies. SPECIAL BENEFIT: Adrenaline helps pep up the heart if a person suffers from shock or collapse, such as in heart failure. Where does the power come to perform these functions? From foods that are given to the adrenal glands!

How to Adjust Your Adrenal Glands Clock. The glands, themselves, are rich in Vitamin C. This means you should drink lots of fresh fruit juices and also eat lots of fresh fruits. The same applies to vitamin- and mineral-rich vegetables and their juices. Here are some suggestions:

Adrenal Protein Punch. The adrenals need protein which combines (in metabolized amino acids) with Vitamin C from vegetable juices to help promote a natural alertness and vigor. Try this healthful punch:

Mix two tablespoons of soybean powder in one glass of freshly squeezed vegetable juice. Add one-half teaspoon of honey. Stir vigorously. Drink slowly.

Benefit: The protein and the vitamins work to help boost a healthful blood sugar level to soothe nervous disorders. The adrenals soak up these nutrients and work to issue the nerve-building hormones.

Whole Grain Breakfast. Europeans have long put their trust in a whole grain breakfast. The benefit of the following "Whole Grain Breakfast" is in the natural supply of healthful carbohydrates from the outer husks of non-processed grains. These feed the adrenals and promote a smooth-flowing blood sugar level and a tranquil emotional level.

    1 tablespoon whole flaxseed
    2 tablespoons wheat bran
    4 tablespoons whole buckwheat grains
    4 tablespoons whole oats
    1 cup vegetable broth

Soak all grains in the vegetable broth overnight. In the morning, warm up, stir well, add honey to taste, and then eat this Whole Grain Breakfast. *Gland Benefits:* The rich supply of natural sugar, healthful B-complex vitamins, as well as many minerals, form a natural alkalizing benefit to the entire system. The adrenal glands will then absorb this treasure of alkalizing nutrients and work efficiently to issue forth the steady "ticking" of rhythmic hormones for much of the day. This will help give you a steady balance and enable you to work smoothly and meet minor crises with youthful emotional-physical strength.

6. *The Pancreas Gland.* Located below the stomach, this is a large, long organ (called the "sweetbread" in animals). Specifically, it is located behind the lower part of the stomach; hence, its value in the digestive process that determines youthful health. *Pancreas Gland Hormone Produced:* Insulin is the hormone that regulates the use of sugar in the body. The bulk of the pancreas is concerned with the manufacture of digestive juices, especially enzymes, which empty out of the pancreas through the common bile duct from the liver. NOTE: Insulin is the spark that ignites the fire for burning sugars and starches and turning them into youthful energy and body heat. Without insulin in balanced amounts, the blood is unable to convert sugar to its needs. Results? The blood cannot *burn* the sugar to produce needed energy; the sugar lies unused in the bloodstream. This leads to an accumulation of sugars and starches that lead to overweight and problems of diabetes. So we see that insulin, a power hormone, must be produced in healthful quantities to maintain weight health and resist problems of diabetes.

How to Adjust Your Pancreas Gland Clock. In brief, *eliminate all white sugar from your diet.* It is the excess amount of sugar intake that causes malfunctioning of your Pancreas Gland Clock. Here are other suggestions:

1. Avoid caffeine-containing products, such as soft drinks, cocoa, chocolate, tea, coffee, etc. These interfere with sugar metabolization and figure into the disruption of this gland clock.

2. To help regulate sugar metabolization, frequently partake of high-protein meals; in between meals, eat protein snacks. SUGGESTION: Try non-processed cheese, eggs, beans, nuts, and organic meats for your protein.

3. Go easy on any food that contains white flour or white sugar, and try to eliminate it entirely from your diet.

4. For healthful starches (yes, there are healthful starches), try completely whole grain cereals and vegetables such as potatoes and beans. NOTE: This type of complete and healthful starch will be taken up by the pancreas to enable it to work smoothly to issue a steady supply of rhythmic-pouring insulin.

5. It means you should omit candy, pastries, cake, soft drinks, white bread, noodles, spaghetti, and macaroni—no adding of white sugar to anything at all! Prudent avoidance of white sugar and flour helps adjust your Pancreas Gland Clock to bring about a healthful metabolization, an enzymatic rhythm that, in turn, leads to a hormone rhythm.

HINTS: To keep your Pancreas Gland Clock well-adjusted, select wholesome, natural foods which have no additives. Occasionally, go on a raw vegetable juice fast to cleanse out your system of toxic debris and enable your pancreas (and other gland clocks) to enjoy a peaceful rest in your body. Just one day on a juice fast and your gland clocks will once again exhibit smooth functioning power.

7. *The Female Sex Glands or Ovaries.* Located in the lower abdomen of the female, these glands are involved in reproduction. *Ovaries Glands Hormones Produced:* Both estrogen and progesterone are issued forth from these glands to control the development of the female sex characteristics and female reproduction. They also exert a strong influence on a woman's emotional and physical life. These female sex glands are also "influenced" by hormones from the pituitary and thyroid glands, attesting to the fact that all of the body's gland clocks tick forth in unified harmony. All of them require careful nourishment and care to promote youthful health. If one is out of order, the other clocks become run down, too.

How to Adjust the Ovaries Glands Clock. Healthful hormones come ticking forth in the presence of a good protein program, modest fat, and low carbohydrates. The emphasis here is on natural hormone foods. Adulterated or treated foods will introduce a large excess of sugar and starch which will cause disarray between the glands. A woman with healthy glands will be able to meet the challenges of daily living and have emotional-physical health.

In particular, the ovaries require nourishment from Vitamins A and C, and also Vitamin E. SUGGESTIONS: Lots of yellow and green vegetables and rich-colored fruits, as well as whole grain products.

"Forever Young" Female Tonic: In a glass of freshly squeezed vegetable juice, stir two tablespoons of wheat germ oil. Stir vigorously and drink. The combination of Vitamins A, B-complex, as well as precious Vitamin E, will work to rejuvenate the ovaries and help promote a healthful rhythm of female hormones—to help keep a woman forever young, forever female!

7-A. *The Male Sex Glands or Testes, and the Prostate Gland.* The testes or male sex glands are located in the scrotal sac, which hangs just below the pelvic area in the male. They influence male characteristics and sperm development. Located just below the bladder and encircling the urethra where it exits from the bladder, the prostate gland influences lubrication of spermatozoa and controls discharge of seminal fluid during copulation, as well as regulating urine discharge. Since it is located immediately in front of the rectum, it is influenced by foods eaten and passed off. *Male Sex Gland Hormone Produced:* The hormone of testosterone, manufactured in the male sex glands or testes, is often regarded as the key to halting premature aging. Stimulation of testosterone production may well bring about a postponement of premature aging. This hormone also helps rebuild flabby muscles, prevents the prostate from enlarging and keeps it healthy, stimulates sluggish brain cells, nourishes the heart muscles, and brings about renewed muscle tone throughout the body (including the muscles of the abdomen and bladder). This may well be the key to the male fountain of youth—the testosterone hormone manufactured by the testes.

How to Adjust the Testes and Prostate Gland Clock. Unsaturated fatty acids found in egg, rice bran oil, sunflower seed oil, cottonseed oil, wheat germ oil, and other vegetable and cereal oils, help to "lubricate" the Prostate Gland Clock and stimulate the testes to manufacture youth-building testosterone. NOTE: This means it is best to eliminate the hard or hydrogenated fats and replace them with these unsaturated fatty acids.

Sarsaparilla: Hope for Hormone Rhythm. Herbal healers and many modern scientists have found that a highly concentrated extract of the sarsaparilla plant has not only one hormone but three— progesterone, cortin, and testosterone. This is a botanical and all-natural source of hormones which may be beneficial for the male. Your herbalist or herbal pharmacist should be able to give you powdered sarsaparilla from which you may make a cup of tea and drink daily.

Magnesium Helps Correct Hormone Rhythm. One mineral, magnesium, has been successfully used in treating prostate troubles, including enlarged prostate and poor male hormone rhythm. In one report[2] some 10 out of 12 males given magnesium tablets were relieved of prostate disorder; furthermore, the doctors reported an

---

[2]*Equilbre Mineral et Santé,* Joseph Favier, M.D., Librairie le Francois, Paris.

adjustment of the Prostate Gland Clock and a feeling of youthful energy in the men. Others who took magnesium in supplement form had not developed prostate-hormone irregularities for years. These men, reportedly, exhibited youthful energy and vitality because this mineral, magnesium, helped boost their healthful glandular rhythm.

Vitamin E: Hormone Tonic. Vitamin E has also been hailed as a miraculous hormone energizer which "oils" the male sex gland clocks, helping them to issue forth their gushing springs of youth-building hormones. Vitamin E is available in capsule as well as liquid supplementation at pharmacies, health food shops, and herbalists.

Glands: Gateway to Hormone Health and Happiness.

Everything we think, do, or eat, has its influence upon the *core* of our existence—our endocrine glandular system. In some situations, one or two reported hormone food programs helped wind up the gland clocks and kept them functioning smoothly with their steady outpouring of youth-building hormones. In other situations, an entire corrective hormone food health program was required to help maintain a natural balance within the system to then facilitate a steady issuing of the rhythm of life: hormones. In *all* situations, the emphasis is upon a *natural* way of life.

With the ever increasing understanding of glands and their youth-promoting hormones, we may well be on the threshold of a new era—the Hormone Age. Indeed, if there is a secret of staying young, it is basically the secret of maintaining healthy and well-regulated hormones. The Fountain of Youth lies within your own body in the form of seven basic glands. When you are able to adjust your "biological gland clocks" properly through all-natural means, when you are able to benefit from an internal "hormone rhythm," you may then hope to enjoy a "feel young for life" treasure of good health.

Highlights of Chapter 1

1. Natural hormone food health programs help wind up, adjust, and tune your biological gland clocks.

2. A healthful 11-Point Natural Hormone Food Program serves as the foundation for "winding up" your gland clocks.

3. Each of the body's seven endocrine glands can be individually adjusted to create hormone rhythm and healthy harmony.

4. Emphasize non-processed and natural hormone foods as a means of building your "fountain of youth" through well-nourished and invigorated endocrine glands.

5. Your "fountain of youth" is within your own body in the form of seven basic glands described in this chapter.

2

How Certain Hormone Foods Help Create Natural Digestive Hormones: The Key to Youthful Health at All Ages

Fruits that ripen naturally on sun-nourished trees, offer a treasure of nutrients that become "hormone food" for your digestive glands. These fruits are especially beneficial in that they provide a source of substances needed by digestive glands as "nourishment" and "fuel" in order to provide the hormones needed for metabolization and assimilation. Tree-ripened fruits are a special source of nutrients for the digestive glands. They offer a bonus of natural substances that help to put a feeling of youth-plus into the digestive glands.

The miracle of digestive hormones is seen when we learn that the stomach has some 35 million "glands"—each of which needs its supply of nourishment in order to produce the valuable hormones needed for digestion and assimilation. In tree-ripened fruits, we have a veritable treasure house of these valuable "gland foods."

How Hormone Foods Rejuvenate Digestive Gland Power

When tree-growing fruits are allowed to ripen by natural means, they become enriched with a prime source of vitamins, minerals, enzymes, and proteins, that serve to energize and revitalize the digestive glands, helping them issue forth the valuable hormones that are vital for the assimilation of foods. When these fruits are

31

nature-ripened on tree tops, they often develop a natural supply of carbohydrates or easily digested fruit sugars. This is the key to digestive gland youth.

Secret Gland Food in Tree-Ripened Fruits. When nature ripens tree-top fruits, she brings about an activity of starch-splitting enzymes in those fruits. The starch is nature-converted into healthful fruit sugar. This natural change of texture and flavor accounts for the good taste of these tree-ripened fruits. When you eat these fruits, your digestive glands welcome their nutrients because their natural fruit sugars provide a powerhouse of energy. The glands then use these invert sugars to promote a normal metabolism and an issuance of digestive hormones. Digestive glands favor the excellent utilization of tree-ripened fruit sugars, the softness of the fiber, the bulky residues produced by pectins, the alkalizing action on the glands, themselves, and a slow release of natural carbohydrates.

Tree-ripened fruits offer these benefits to the digestive glands so they can use absorbed nutrients to issue forth the precious hormones which are then used for assimilation of other ingested foods. You are as young and healthy as your digestive system! The secret to digestive youth often lies in the secret of these tree-ripened "gland foods." Here are other benefits to your digestive gland system as offered by tree-ripened fruits:

1. *Vitamin A Helps Feed Digestive Glands.* Tree-ripened fruits offer a splendid source of Vitamin A, which is then used by the digestive glands to issue hormones to soothe the skin and mucous membranes of the body organs.

2. *A Treasure of Hormone Energizers.* Tree-ripened fruits introduce a set of other vitamins such as thiamine, riboflavin, niacin, Vitamin C, all entering into the glandular metabolization to issue forth an energetic flow of hormones. The hormones, themselves, are made of these nutrients and can function with energy solely according to the intake of such energizers. Tree-ripened fruits offer a treasure house of these hormone fluids.

3. *Hormone Foods Enable Digestive Glands to Boost Blood Cell Health.* The digestive glands have the responsibility of facilitating iron absorption, and then building the red blood cells. A look and feel of youth depends upon a healthy bloodstream. The digestive glands need the high iron content found in tree-ripened fruits. These glands then work to metabolize the iron and issue forth those hormones that work to promote the rich hemoglobin and red coloring that indicates good blood cell health. *NOTE:* Prunes,

apricots, and peaches are the *three* highest sources of iron amongst the family of tree-ripened fruits. These *three* fruits are extremely beneficial to digestive glands because of their need for spark plugs in order to manufacture hormones which then help boost blood cellular health.

4. *Digestive Gland Youth Is Energized by Hormone Foods.* These tree-ripened fruits are often called "sunshine youth" fruits. This is a benefit well-earned because tree-ripening fruits drink in the sunshine until they reach full maturity; they are then harvested with all the goodness and multiplicity of nutrient values that are sealed in and preserved by nature, to be released to your digestive glands when the fruit is eaten.

Source of Digestive Youth Feeling. Tree-ripened fruits have an exceptionally high content of quickly assimilable fruit sugars, due in large part to this complete ripening. They become a source of quick energy for the digestive organs, and stimulate the digestive glands to issue forth the youth-healthy hormones needed for good assimilation.

5. *Hormone Foods That Promote Digestive Balance.* The nutrients in these fruits are taken by the digestive glands to help promote natural regularity. The glands are energized by the nutrients to issue forth hormones to assimilate food into natural, soft bulk. The hormones then work to create the good muscle tone needed to provide healthful body elimination.

Active Principle in Fruits. Tree-ripened fruits are among the very few natural hormone foods with an active principle that is needed by digestive glands to regulate the actions of the large intestine. It is this principle that awakens a sluggish digestive gland system to issue forth healthful hormones that promote digestive balance and help ease the problem of constipation.

6. *Natural Stimulation of Gastric Secretion.* Tree-ripened fruits promote an increased salivary flow, which is attributed to direct sensitization of the secretory nerve endings in the salivary glands. This action, in turn, stimulates the digestive glands to cause an increase in gastric secretion and promote a gentle and prolonged hormone rhythm that facilitates basic digestion. *The glands determine the effectiveness of digestion!* These glands need the substances in tree-ripened fruits from which they create the hormones to promote healthful assimilation of foods. And it is the assimilation that determines the health and the "forever young" feeling of the entire person. All depend upon healthy and youthfully nourished digestive glands.

7. *Hormone-Food Nourished Glands Promote Youthful Digestive Hormones.* Tree-ripened fruits stimulate the rhythmic flow of hor mones from nourished glands. This helps bring warmth and a roseate outlook to the person; this increases the flow of the digestive juices and helps promote a look and feeling of internal youth.

In Review: Tree-ripened fruits offer the "food" for digestive glands to enable them to issue forth digestive hormones. Fruits provide a pectin and delicate fiber network that feed the digestive gland system. The natural fruit sugars of tree-ripened hormone foods are especially beneficial to the glands *because they are protein sparing*—an added benefit. The glands utilize the fruit sugars *without* excessive use of protein, so that there is a healthful digestive balance. The tree-ripened fruits offer these benefits to your glands and help bring about youthful digestion.

How a Hormone Food Program Promoted "Young Again" Digestion

Susan E., at age 46, experienced recurring problems with her digestion. She envied the gusto with which her youngsters ate and subsequently digested their foods. Conversely, much of what Susan E. would eat remained in her stomach "feeling like a clump of hard dough," with occasional stomach spasms, twisting and churning pains that were most pronounced in the middle of the night (when metabolism is at a very low rate and undigested food remains in a painful stomach bulk), and also an embarrassing feeling of irregularity.

The Laxative Habit Tormented Digestive Glands. Susan E. fell into the laxative habit, trying candy, chocolate-flavored cathartics, salts, liquids, and "milks" that caused such colonic upheaval, she felt worse than ever before. Whatever she ate left her with a feeling of discomfort. Now she felt enslaved to the laxative habit.

Dietary Adjustment and Tree-Top Fruits Help Ease Symptoms. Unable to eat irritating foods, Susan E. made adjustments and eliminated items that were made of bleached white flour and white sugar. She found that tree-top fruits were soothing. She followed this suggested hormone food program to help nourish her weak digestive glands:

BEGIN MEAL WITH FRESH TREE-TOP FRUIT: On an empty stomach, Susan E. took a fruit salad composed of freshly sliced and uncooked apples, bananas, peaches, sun-dried prunes, and seasonal berries. *Nothing else.* NOTE: She would take this raw tree-top fruit salad about 60 minutes *before* a meal. *Benefit:* The weary digestive glands soaked up the treasure of nutrients in the fruit and were able to stimulate a healthful flow of stomach hormones, which, in turn, prepared Susan's digestive system for the food to follow. Now she could enjoy healthfully prepared foods with less of the after-meal discomfort.

BANANAS: KEY TO REGULARITY. Susan E. sought to establish regularity *without* the use of harsh laxatives or cathartics. She found that tree-ripened bananas are especially beneficial to the sluggish digestive glands. Daily, she would eat several whole bananas—nothing else at that particular time. *Benefit:* The natural laxative properties of the banana stimulated the digestive glands to issue forth hormones to promote normal functioning of the colon. The fine fibrous cellular material served to help correct Susan's constipation. Her digestive hormones took up the non-irritating fiber, which was then used to give bulk to intestinal residues. *How Hormones Helped:* The digestive hormones brought the banana pectin to the intestinal region; the pectin is water absorbent and therefore expands, lubricating the intestinal wall. The hormones were gently aroused by tree-ripened fruit sugars to promote this internal rhythmic sensation. This hormone food, bananas, proved to be the key to Susan's regularity.

BERRIES BOOSTED GLANDULAR VIGOR. Susan E. then began eating a bowl of freshly washed, tree-ripened seasonal berries almost every single day. The berries contained ingredients that enabled the digestive glands to cause a flow of minerals into the bloodstream, thereby enriching the power of the hormone rivers of life. The glands needed the iron in the tree-ripened berries to cause regeneration of hemoglobin, working together with niacin and Vitamin C, to promote healthful mucous secretion and facilitate absorption of "nourishment" for the body's organs. Once the hormone rhythm was established, Susan E. was able to look and feel young with a healthful digestive system. Tree-ripened fruits were "nature's medicines" for her glandular system.

How to Feed Your Glands with Hormone-Producing Tree-Ripened Fruits

You can help nourish your glands by feeding them a wide variety of seasonal and fresh, raw tree-ripened fruits. NOTE: Obtain organic, naturally grown fruits whenever possible. See to it that they are allowed to ripen *naturally* on the tree tops, so that nature brings about the fruit sugar metabolization that offers a treasure of value to the body glands. If you have no choice and obtain fruits grown on chemically fertilized soils, sprayed with harsh insecticides, or picked *before* natural ripening occurs, then you may not experience the maximum benefits. In this case, be sure to wash these fruits under freshly poured and free-flowing cold tap water. Use a fruit or vegetable scrub brush to cleanse out as much of the spray residue as possible. *Peel* these fruits, whenever possible. Nature's protective coating helps keep out much of the spray residue from the fruit pulp beneath.

Here are ways in which you can nourish your digestive glands with tree-ripened fruits:

1. Before your main meal, eat a plate of raw and freshly cut tree-ripened fruits. About 30 to 60 minutes *before* a meal is beneficial, since the fruits need to be metabolized by digestive glands and some time is required. Doing so means that by the time you are ready to eat your meal, your digestive glands will be nourished and issue forth soothing hormones to help boost your powers of assimilation.

2. Once a week, put yourself on a tree-top raw fruit fast! Eat nothing but fresh, raw, tree-top ripened fruit for all of your meals. This is highly beneficial to your digestive glands, since they are now able to work solely with the ingested fruits and without interference of competitive foods. The digestive glands welcome this fasting program with tree-top raw fruits.

3. Occasionally, eat one meal that is exclusively made up of fresh, tree-top raw fruits! This could be an evening meal. It is best to do so during the evening, since your digestive glands will then have the nutrients from fruits to work upon *while you sleep!* A mild metabolism during the night is a healthful media for fruits. You'll awaken in the morning with a "look and feel young" comfort in your digestive system. Your digestive glands have been churning away soothingly throughout the night, issuing forth a treasure of hormones to help you meet the next day with health and happiness.

Tree-Ripened Figs: The Source of Digestive "Gland Power"

Fresh, sun-dried, tree-ripened figs hold the "secret" of digestive gland power. If there is one fruit that should stand out alone in its ability to nourish and rejuvenate digestive glands, it may well be the fig. Hailed among healers for thousands of years, the fig is coming into its own, today, as a miracle source of "gland power." The secret may well be in its method of pollination, which enables its nutrients to slowly give birth and then blossom forth in substances which promote the natural and healthful flow of digestive hormones.

"Forever Young" Glands Through Hormone Foods. As a librarian, Fred T. often remained in the musty archives throughout the day, or even in early evening. His meals were erratic. He looked pale and thin. He felt weak. He displayed the symptoms of premature aging, with recurring sniffles, digestive unrest, embarrassing bouts of prolonged constipation, and recurring colitis. He subsisted on flat-tasting sandwiches made with harsh, white, bleached bread. His health was declining.

Researched Lore of Fruit Medicine! Fred T. was given a research project about fruits. While looking through various books in the library, he learned that figs had been regarded as "medicine" for many, many hundreds of centuries. He read how the ancient Greeks in Crete, back in 1500 B.C., looked upon the fig as a source of energy and youthful power. Further readings revealed that this tree-ripened fruit could increase the strength of young people, preserve the elderly in better health, reportedly smooth out wrinkled skin, and even promote a youthful strength. (The Greek athletes and champions were often given meals consisting solely of fresh tree-ripened figs.) Many more health benefits were attributed to figs. *Fred T. discovered that this tree-ripened fruit was more than just a food—it was a natural medicine for the glands!*

A Fig Fast Program Helps Enrich Fred's Gland Health. He followed a folklore hormone food program that called for spending one day a week with tree-ripened figs! He ate little else on that day, except for a raw fruit salad which was seasoned with a mixture of lemon and apple juice for a soothing dressing. The figs that Fred ate during his one-day "fig fast" offered these glandular-boosting bene-fits:

1. Figs worked upon the glands, gently prompting them to provide smooth bulk to work an emollient effect upon the intestine, and help bring about intestinal regularity.

2. Figs gave much valuable Vitamin A as well as thiamine, riboflavin, niacin, plus other nutritives in the B-complex family, to the digestive glands. The glands then used these nutrients to manufacture a steady supply of hormones. The hormones, themselves, need these nutrients to promote body rhythm.

3. The figs offered the glands a healthful source of energy; quickly assimilable fruit sugars such as dextrose and levulose—found mostly in tree-ripened fruits—energized and alerted the glands, helping them function more adequately.

4. Figs helped establish a natural and healthful acid-alkaline balance. The digestive glands need the nutrients in such hormone foods as tree-ripened figs in order to help maintain a normal and healthful alkaline reserve in the body. This meets the challenge of excess acid. NOTE: Tree-ripened figs, and other fruits, help create this valuable alkaline reserve by nourishing digestive glands to issue forth the hormones charged with this responsibility. These hormones then work to create a pool of alkaline reserve that will be rushed to an acid-burning portion of the stomach in a crisis, providing naturally soothing comfort. The *key* to forming this alkaline pool reserve is through tree-ripened fruits, which offer vigor to digestive glands and help create needed hormones to maintain the alkaline reserve. Again, the key is through the source of energy for the glands—tree-ripened fruits, particularly figs.

Fred T. Enjoys Youthful Gland Harmony. By emphasizing figs, as well as other hormone foods, Fred T. could enjoy the benefits of youthful gland harmony. A fountain of soothing hormones now made his skin look better, his energy improved, irregularity was healed, and he walked with a better gait. BUT—the habitual use of artificial foods and processed, pre-packaged meats, as well as chemically treated foods, tended to *block* the full action of the nourished glands. Fred T. enjoyed a *partial* youthful comeback. If he would have followed an all-natural program, he might have been able to benefit from a well-nourished glandular system. You are as healthy as your glands! Nourish them properly and completely and you enjoy more wholesome health. Nourish them partially, as did Fred T., and you enjoy only a partial restoration of glandular health.

Tree-Ripened Fruits—Hormone Food for Your Glands

By eating these fresh, *raw* tree-ripened fruits, you help provide food for your glands. You give your glands the health-boosting vital nutritive elements which they use for digestive function as well as for the manufacture of valuable youth-building hormones. Here are some tree-ripened fruits which are prime sources of nutritive treasures for the glands.

Bananas	Cherries
Dates	Papayas
Figs	Apples
Raisins	Plums
Grapes	Apricots
Prunes	Melons
Pears	Avocados
Oranges	Pomegranates
Grapefruits	Tangerines
Pineapples	Strawberries
Lemons	Blackberries
Limes	Huckleberries

You will probably find other tree-ripened fruits at your local outlet. Select those that are in season, that are organic (if possible) and of a fresh and healthy look. MOST IMPORTANT: The fruits should have been allowed to ripen full term on the tree top. This has enabled nature to prepare them with fully developed nutrients to feed and nourish your glandular system. An organic food outlet usually has naturally tree-ripened fruits and should be your best source of wholesome foods.

Six Gland-Rejuvenating Benefits of Hormone Foods

Nearly all organically grown, tree-ripened fruits will offer these six basic gland-rejuvenating benefits:

1. The fruits contain seed and fibre bulk in combination with a natural solvent in the liquid that is believed vital for digestive glands to promote intestinal regularity.

2. The fruits contain a high excess alkalinity of ash that enables the digestive glands to promote a youthful acid-alkaline balance in the digestive system, often the key to youthful health.

3. The tree-ripened fruits are known for containing special protein-digesting enzymes that liberate amino acids which are eagerly absorbed by the glands as "fuel" for manufacturing hormones.

4. The fruits contain many minerals, such as calcium, iron, potassium, magnesium, copper, and iodine—all needed by the glands which control hormones that create strong bones, rich blood, healthy and happy nerves, healing of wounds, and liver and skin-cell metabolism.

5. The fruits contain nutrients that are needed by the glands to assist in the production of hemoglobin and promote cell oxygenation—the very foundation of hormone rhythm and prolonged youth.

6. The fruits are prime sources of vitamins needed to create cells and tissues, build up immunity to infections, and resist the ravages of unnecessary and premature aging; most valuable, the glands metabolize these vitamins from tree-ripened fruits into principles that go into the hormones . . . the smooth-flowing rivers of life.

Remember—nature has created tree-growing fruits so that the natural method of ripening could promote a "sun cooked" storehouse of valuable nutrients, as well as fruit sugars, which form the energy base for the hormones, themselves. These tree-ripened nutrients are the life's blood of the fruit—and the very life's blood of the digestive glands. Just as they nourish the fruit to promote a healthy, sun-washed life, so can the sheer goodness in the fruit awaken and alert the body glands to a healthful hormonal rhythm. The life of the body's glands may well be in the life of the tree-ripened fruits of nature—the source of life and health!

In Review

1. Tree-ripened fruits are special sources of nutrients that feed and nourish the body's digestive glands, alerting them to a "forever young" hormone-sparked digestion.

2. Tree-ripened fruits offer a set of seven special benefits to the digestive glandular network.

3. Susan E. enjoyed a "young again" digestive system by nourishing her glands with a simple and tasty tree-top fruit program.

4. Feed your glands by following the simple three-step outlined program that used wholesome, tree-ripened fruits.

5. Tree-ripened figs stand out as one single source of digestive gland power.

6. Fred T. partially restored youthful gland harmony with figs.

7. Keep in mind the six basic gland-rejuvenating benefits of tree-ripened fruits.

3

How "Magic" Plants Nourish the Glands to Produce Hormones for Youthful Skin and Hair

        Sea plants harvested from the depths of the briny ocean·offer a buried treasure of minerals that help nourish your thyroid gland and prompt the stimulation of a hormone that promotes a "forever young" skin and healthy scalp. The ocean is one of the richest sources of minerals in the world. Sea vegetation is especially high in these gland-feeding minerals because of the rhythmic process of soil erosior. Because of overcropping and land erosion, land mineral-rich soil is constantly being washed into the seas of the world, bringing about further enrichment. The benei here is that the total mineral supply of sea vegetation is some 20 times higher than any land-grown food. It is reported that some 22 minerals are found in sea plants, as well as beneficial quantities of vitamins and some forms of protein. These hormone foods converge together to provide nourishment for the entire network of glands, but in particular they offer *iodine* to the *thyroid gland,* which is then able to manufacture the *thyroxine hormone*—the little "beauty stream" that works to keep your skin and hair looking healthy and youthful.

    How Ocean-Plant Hormone Foods Nourish your Thyroid Gland— Key to Healthy Skin and Hair. These ocean plants feed upon the rain waters which have washed mineral-rich opsoi. into pouring rivers and streams. The plants become rich sources oi such soluble minerals, which have been eroded and leached rom soil, rock and forest humus. In particular, the plants are the prime sources o

41

iodine—the one mineral that is food for the thyroid, more than for any other gland. The thyroid gland then takes up the treasure of iodine, together with a special nutrient known as di-iodotyrosine. The thyroid gland takes this ingredient, converts it to thyroxine, and the hormone is then sent gushing into the bloodstream.

Hormone Food Boosts Skin Youth. Thyroxine is sent to nourish and rejuvenate the millions of capillary blood vessels, lymph vessels, nerve endings, and sebaceous glands. Thyroxine prompts these sebaceous glands to secrete a skin-youth substance called sebum that helps keep the skin and hair looking alive, firm, and healthful.

Thyroxine further nourishes the subcutaneous tissue, feeding the tiny fat cells beneath. *Benefit:* The thyroxine hormone, well-nourished by iodine and other minerals from ocean plants, plumps up these tiny fat cells, helping to soften the contours of the body, serving as a firm and youthful cushior between muscles and skin.

Hormone Food Promotes Skin Rejuvenation. The thyroxine hormone further works to stimulate the skin follicles to extract water, salt, and waste substances from the capillaries, and releases them at the skin surfaces through tiny openings or pores. It is this rhythmic process that sends a rich supply of hormone nourishment to the surface beneath the skin to help promote skin rejuvenation.

Hormone Food Boosts Hair Youth. In many reported cases, the increased intake of iodine fed the thyroid gland so it could manufacture a steady supply of thyroxine, which helped boost the health and youth of hair. An iodine deficiency often manifests itself first in premature graying, dry hair, stringy hair, lacklustre quality, and unnatural hair loss. By regulating the "thyroid clock" with adequate amounts of iodine so it can issue a steady rhythmic ticking flow of thyroxine, the hair follicles receive nourishment to help boost hair youth.

Minerals from ocean plants prompt the rhythm of thyroxine, which is sent streaming into the circulatory system to feed the hair follicles (hair roots) and penetrate into the layer of fat beneath the scalp. The thyroxine nourishes the tiny oil glands found near the surface of the scalp, feeding these wellsprings so they can then issue forth their substances, which influence the health and quality of hair.

Iodine, in particular, is needed to enter into the composition of thyroxine, which is "food" for the scalp roots. Thyroxine works with body proteins to metabolize other nutrients to help feed the delicate and microscopic hair follicles. *Benefit:* The thyroxine hormone, sparked with its supply of iodine and the other vitamins-minerals-proteins from ocean plants, enters into the epidermis and the fibrous, living tissues, as well as the hair follicles and nerve endings, feeding the *papilla* (a small bulb-like root from which hair is grown and youthfully maintained) and nourishing the tiny little bulb so it can send forth the substances needed to help promote youthful and healthy hair. This miracle of nature is made possible by feeding the thyroid gland a good supply of iodine, such as found in the rich treasure house of the vegetation beneath the briny depths of the world's oceans and seas.

Four Hormone Foods That Offer "Skin-Hair Youth" Through Feeding of Your Thyroid Gland

The use of ocean plants has been known for some 5,000 years. It is believed to have originated in the Orient, where seaweed was long regarded as an exquisite delicacy and even offered as a sacred sacrifice to the gods. The harvesting of marine crops has taken place for hundreds of centuries, and it continues in our modern times. Diving girls from seaside villages swim in the gardens of the oceans where they bring up different varieties of sea plants, which are treasure houses of minerals, notably of iodine, an ideal hormone food! Here are four ocean plants that are available in many health food stores, herbal pharmacies, as well as special diet shops:

1. *Seaweed—Hormone Food for Skin and Hair.* A popular variety that originates in Japan is a thin sheet of seaweed. It may be crumbled and sprinkled on food, or it may be toasted by holding it over a low flame for just a few seconds. It is a good source of minerals that are absorbed by the thyroid gland to manufacture skin-hair food, via the hormone thyroxine. Seaweed from Japan is also used as an ingredient in packaged relishes, cakes, desserts, and beverages. Many of these products are available in natural health store outlets.

2. *Kelp—The Hormone-Boosting Sea Salt.* Kelp is a powdered form of an ocean plant which grows in the Pacific, along the Atlantic coast, as well as in some of the oceans in the Southern hemisphere. Kelp is a prime source of the hormone food *iodine.* This mineral prompts the thyroid gland to manufacture sufficient amounts of iodine, which is then used in the manufacture of thyroxine. *Special Benefit:* Kelp offers a type of iodine that issues a rhythmic and

steady hormone flow to help keep the hair and skin in a regulated form of health.

Five Hormone-Stimulating Benefits of Kelp. Iodine from kelp stimulates the thyroid gland to pour forth hormones which offer these basic benefits:

Firms Up Skin. Iodine in kelp has a rhythmic benefit on the thyroid gland, helping to tone up flabby skin, smooth out furrows and wrinkles, and diminish unnecessary amounts of skin-fat accumulations.

Stimulates Membranes and Lymphatics. An invigorated and youthfully stimulated, kelp-nourished thyroid gland sends thyroxine to help alert the sluggish membranes and stimulate the health of the lymphatics (similar to blood vessels which collect nutrients to feed the bloodstream as well as the skin-hair network). The result is a healthy skin and healthy hair.

Gently Stimulating and Toning Up. Thyroxine is energized by minerals in kelp to influence the fatty globules and promote a general toning up of the skin and hair.

Boosts Function of Body Organs Through Nourished Thyroid. Iodine in kelp offers a remedial and normalizing benefit to the thyroid, so that the thyroxine "beauty stream" will help to nourish the sensory nerves, arteries, gall bladder, bile ducts, and kidneys. When these other body organs are in smooth hormone-nourished rhythm, the skin and hair show a healthful and youthful lustre.

Internal Cleansing Agent. Kelp minerals spark the rhythmic flow of iodine-rich thyroxine to enter into the valuable process of internal cleansing. As a cleansing agent, iodine-rich thyroxine works to help soothe arterial tension, give tone to the walls of the blood vascular network, and help restore venous-arterial elasticity, thereby aiding the body in building a healthy skin and hair. Kelp may well be the one miracle "hormone food" that builds healthy youth—from the inside out!

How to Use Kelp in Your Hormone Food Program. In its powdered form, available at most health food and special diet shops, kelp is tasteful as a salt substitute. Sprinkle over salads, cottage cheese, on baked potatoes, on meat dishes. *Tip:* Try kelp as a salt substitute when baking bread or cookies.

Other Eating Suggestions: Try kelp in tablet form as a nutritional mineral supplement for your thyroid and other glands. Kelp is also available as a vegetable gelatine for tasty desserts; it is also in flake form to be added to a glass of fresh vegetable juice.

3. *Irish Moss—The Mineral Tonic for a Youthful Thyroid.* This ocean plant, also known as *carrageen,* is a powerhouse of vitamins and minerals that offer one special and unique benefit:

Alkaline Source: The rich alkaline source in Irish Moss makes it a very soothing food that is said to help restore the delicate acid-alkaline balance that enters into the rhythmic flow of thyroxine from the thyroid gland. *Other benefits:* Irish Moss is very low in calories. It also has a preponderance of calcium and phosphorus. These two minerals are regulated by thyroxine to help build strong bone structure, firm up the nerves and skin-hair cellular network, assist in metabolism, and boost the health of the body.

How to Use Irish Moss in Your Hormone Food Program. Available at the aforementioned health shops, Iri,h Moss may be used as a substitute for animal gelatine in jellos, puddings, or custards, and as a thickener in sauces, broths, and soups.

Irish Moss Dessert: Soak one-quarter cup of Irish Moss in cold water about 15 minutes. Now stir in one quart of boiled water. Let simmer until Irish Moss has dissolved. Add the juice of two lemons. Add a quarter teaspoon of cinnamon. Sweeten with natural honey. Strain into molds. Makes a powerhouse of "thyroid food" in the form of an all-natural dessert!

How a "Thyroid Booster Cocktail" Created a "Forever Young" Feeling

Irene T. felt her vitality at a low ebb. Added to the distress were the furrowed wrinkles and crease-lines in her skin that were telltale symptoms of premature aging. Her once-lustrous hair was now "mousey" and gave her a drab, lifeless appearance. Her memory was somewhat hazy, and there were days when her hands and feet felt cold chills, despite the warmth of the climate.

Irene T. developed problems of rough, dry skin, poor hair, together with slow mental-physical responses. She chafed at the thought that she was "getting on in years" because she was in her early 40's, the prime of life.

Low Blood Pressure: Clue to Sluggish Thyroid. During a routine examination, she was told that she had low blood pressure. This offered a clue to a probably sluggish thyroid. Further tests showed that she was very insufficient in iodine. A problem of hypothyroid (low activity) was a basic cause of her premature aging. She embarked upon a simple recommended program—to drink a simple

"Thyroid Booster Cocktail" upon arising. Here's how it is prepared:

THYROID BOOSTER COCKTAIL. Wash two ounces of Irish Moss in cold water. Now put the washed moss into a kettle containing two quarts of freshly poured, cold water. Place over a low fire. Let simmer until reduced to half the amount. Now strain. Irene T. would drink just *one cup* of this Thyroid Booster Cocktail every morning, upon arising. *Benefit:* In the morning when the digestive system is fresh and vital, and there is no other food with which to interfere, the minerals in the Thyroid Booster Cocktail are exceedingly effective in feeding the thyroid gland, helping to manufacture the much needed hormone, thyroxine.

Irene T. continued this hormone food program every single morning up to three weeks, and she then began to feel and look better. In a month, she was well on the way to better recovery. Her skin and hair improved, she had a sparkle in her eyes, her memory was alert, and life was worth living—thanks to the hormone foods that nourished her thyroid gland.

What the Thyroid Booster Cocktail May Do for You

When the thyroid gland is properly nourished so that the thyroxine hormone is sent throughout your body's "beauty stream" to spark the look and feel of youth, using the minerals in the Thyroid Booster Cocktail, here are the benefits you will receive:

1. An alert and nourished thyroid gland will help control vitality and normal body growth processes.

2. The iodine-fed hormone will help protect the body against poisons and injuries.

3. The hormone works to act as an energizer and lubricator, so that the skin and hair look and feel youthfully healthy.

4. The hormone feeds the little "oil glands" beneath the skin surface, helping in their growth and development.

5. Iodine in the Thyroid Booster Cocktail enters into the thyroxine hormone; this living stream helps promote mental agility and normal quick-thinking impulses.

Helps Rejuvenate Entire Body. The ocean-rich treasures of hormone food nutrients in the Thyroid Booster Cocktail work to remake the entire body and mind. It aids in regulating the metabolism (rate at which food is broken down and built into cells), helps use calcium and phosphorus, influences growth, weight, personality, emotions, heartbeat, body reaction to cold and heat (a sluggish thyroid was responsible for Irene's cold hands and feet), improved memory, and the making of red blood corpuscles. Just a minute amount of iodine can offer such rejuvenating benefits, yet the slightest "starvation" may cause much body disharmony. The value of iodine from ocean plants can never be underestimated!

4. *Algae—Source of Youthful Vigor.* Another sea plant, algae, has been found to be a powerhouse of Vitamins A and D, as well as zinc—the mineral that is highly concentrated in the thyroid. A zinc deficiency may cause derangement of the hormonal rhythm. The person may experience disorders of the prostate gland and pancreas, leading to problems of prostatitis as well as diabetes.

Available in thin sheets and, more popularly, as a powder, algae is a seaweed hormone food that offers a treasure trove of zinc as well as iodine, together with a family of nutrients that work to enter into the formation of thyroxine.

Algae with its zinc power may well be the "double energy" source that provides the spark to the iodine-containing thyroxine. In combination, the enrichment process offers a source of "forever young" hormones that go streaming throughout the body, bathing it with an ocean's treasures of minerals and other essential nutrients.

How to Use Algae: Sold in the form of a powder, algae may well be used as a salt substitute. Use it wherever you would use table salt (to be eliminated in your quest for a healthy hormone system) as a flavoring and seasoning agent. *Just one-half teaspoon of algae powder daily helps provide the enrichment needed by the thyroxine to propel itself throughout the body, building a youthful skin and a healthy hair-growing scalp.*

How "Thyroid Nourishment" Offered a "Feel Young for Life" Benefit

In a reported program[1], the boosting of the thyroid gland by feeding it iodine in supplement form, was able to provide a "feel young for life" benefit in a number of persons. The "miracle" of this rejuvenation is that the basic program called for stimulation of the sluggish thyroid and little else. Here are the reported case histories:

---

[1]Cases cited in speech before the American College of Endocrinology and Nutrition in May, 1966.

Simple Hormone Food Supplement Makes Mrs. R. Young Again. At 64, Mrs. Doris R. was bedridden and in a state of more than just semi-coma; she reportedly was the recipient of the last rites! Her problem was discovered to be that of being a myxedematous female (suffering from a thyroid deficiency) that was symptomatic by her lifeless skin and patchy hair. Immediately, Mrs. R. was given a simple food supplement—one-quarter grain iodine together with Brewer's Yeast (rich in B-complex vitamins).

Bounces Back to Second Youth. This simple thyroid-boosting action that used a simple but all-natural food supplement helped Mrs. R. bounce back to a second youth. The reported improvements: her dead skin peeled away to show new and youthful skin, her white hair became streaked with black, furthermore, her mental faculties returned. She was now in a healthful and "rejuvenated" second youth! All this when her thyroid was nourished with iodine supplements and boosters of Brewer's Yeast.

Hormone Food Promotes Miracle Recovery for Attorney. Mr. L., an attorney, had been forced to retire because of high blood pressure, poor circulation, elevated cholesterols, occasional heart irregularity (missed beats), and poor vision. He was also some 15 pounds underweight (a symptom of an iodine-starved thyroid). Mr. L. was a championship bridge player, but his memory had become so bad that he could not remember what day it was, much less the suits of the cards.

Treatment: Power of Iodine. The treatment called for iodine supplementation—little else, except for a return to more natural and wholesome hormone foods. It sounds simple, but it was reportedly so effective that within six months, his blood pressure returned to normal, his skin and hair improved, his memory was youthful, and he was playing bridge again. Just a few hormone foods with a minute amount of iodine made all the difference between premature aging and effervescent youth!

HOW TO USE B-COMPLEX VITAMINS TO BOOST ACTION OF IODINE. The "secret" of this success is to combine both iodine supplements with the B-complex vitamins through Brewer's yeast. There is a biochemical rationale for this joint therapy. Several of the B-complex vitamins in Brewer's Yeast (riboflavin, niacin, thiamine, and others) are concerned with transport of oxygen within the cell. Iodine works to help thyroxine step up oxidation. Iodine needs the B-complex vitamins in Brewer's Yeast to help prevent loss of energy waste.

HOW B-COMPLEX VITAMINS GIVE PLUS BENEFITS TO IODINE. Iodine alone, in the form of ocean plants, does cause an improvement in metabolism, but its benefits are boosted with the use of Brewer's Yeast. When taken in combination, Vitamin B-complex in Brewer's Yeast works to cause an electron transfer to release useful energy intra-cellularly and boost the thyroid into a healthful rhythm.

A NOURISHED THYROID HELPS EXTEND THE LIFESPAN. It is reported[2] that a well-nourished thyroid helps resist the problems of premature aging, and also helps regulate the process of atherosclerosis. (A form of hardening of the arteries in which the inner lining is involved as a result of fat deposits in it; this is regarded as a forerunner of heart trouble.) A nourished thyroid may well help control the formation of such problems and extend the lifespan.

There is much evidence of a decrease in thyroxine production and utilization with aging, even though laboratory findings may remain within the normal range.

HOW OCEAN PLANTS STIMULATE A SLUGGISH THYROID TO PROMOTE A HEALTHY SKIN-HAIR LIFESPAN. The minerals in ocean plants promote a rhythm of thyroxine which washes throughout the body. This hormone helps in the metabolism of fats and keeps the biological clock ticking away in a steady balance. Faulty lipid (fat) metabolism may lead to the unhealthy deposit of fats on the artery walls; when this happens, the metabolic process goes awry and the skin-hair and health lifespan simultaneously begin to decline. The use of iodine food supplements together with Brewer's Yeast, and the use of the various available ocean plants, may well offer the hormone foods that are needed by the thyroid gland to keep the body looking and feeling well.

Benefits of a Nourished Thyroid: Ocean plants that feed the thyroid with a treasure of vitamins and minerals, offer these benefits: easing problems of nervousness, and depression, soothing the irritated body and mind, energizing the system, promoting a comfortable warmth in hands and feet, improving poor breathing, helping to promote healthful sleep, and improving memory.

The Magic Ingredient in Ocean Plants. One unique hormone food ingredient is that of mannitol—a natural sugar (which does not increase body blood sugar) which is taken up by the thyroid gland

---

[2]James C. Wren, M.D., *Journal of the American Geriatric Society,* January, 1971.

and used as an energizer to send a rich stream of thyroxine into the delicate ducts and tubules leading to the skin-scalp surface. This helps nourish the network of blood vessels that control the health of both the skin and scalp. *Mannitol* is the natural energizer that awakens the thyroid, enters into the composition of thyroxine, and promotes a "look-feel young" appearance of skin and scalp . . . and body and mind!

OTHER SOURCES OF IODINE. While ocean plants are a prime source of iodine, there are other food sources. These include salmon, dark molasses, watercress, sardines (excellent source), eggs, oatmeal, potato with skin, and milk.

GARLIC: PRIME VEGETABLE SOURCE. Of all the vegetables, *garlic* is the richest source of iodine. You might make it a culinary rule of thumb to eat diced, *raw* garlic with raw vegetable salads as a means of boosting your iodine intake and nourishing your thyroid.

SELECT ORGANIC FOODS. Normally, plants absorb iodine from the soil in which it is present. Iodine is also abundantly available in milk, when the mineral is also present in the soil the cows feed upon. Organic soils that are "fed" iodine-rich fertilizers offer healthful organic vegetables as well as fruits. It is best to obtain organic foods as much as possible so the iodine content is not leached out or chemically treated. Wherever possible, buy seafoods, as well as your ocean plants, from a health food or organic food outlet that offers items from *sewage-free ocean waters.*

Special Suggestion: Obtain organic *salt-water fish* varieties, which have a higher supply of iodine than fresh-water fish.

Ocean Plants Are a Prime Source of Thyroid Food. Iodine in seaweeds is in the form of a natural balance, as it occurs in the thyroid gland. It is almost as if nature gave the ocean plants its own thyroxine hormone. This is the reason why iodine from ocean plants is so effective, because it is almost identical to the same form as in the thyroid gland. In your hormone food program to help nourish your skin-hair and body network through an alert and well-nourished thyroid gland, ocean plants should stand out as the prime all-natural source—a youth gift from the sea.

Main Points

1. To promote a healthy skin and hair-growing scalp, feed your thryoid with an abundant supply of iodine from ocean plants.
2. A nourished thyroid gland sends forth thyroxine, the "beauty

stream" hormone that feeds the millions of skin-scalp outlets to promote a healthful and youthful appearance.

3. Four ocean plants are available for thyroid gland feeding.

4. An Irish Moss Dessert makes a powerhouse of "thyroid food" in a delicious, all-natural dessert.

5. Irene T. experienced a marvelous rejuvenation with a simple and all-natural Thyroid Booster Cocktail in the morning. The wonder food ingredients offer five special benefits to promote healthful living.

6. A combination of iodine supplements with simple Brewer's Yeast helped Mrs. R. bounce back to a second youth.

7. Iodine supplements with natural hormone foods promoted miracle youth recovery for an attorney, Mr. L., and made him feel young again.

8. To help boost body health, establish the glandular clock rhythm by feeding natural iodine to the thyroid gland—the key to a perpetual feeling of youth!

4

How Natural Hormones Help
Ease Arthritic Distress
That Ages a Person

Mineral hormones in fresh fruits, vegetables, and dairy products have the power to stimulate the adrenal glands to issue forth a healthful supply of natural ACTH and cortisone hormone, that offer hope for those distressed by arthritic-rheumatic discomforts. These mineral hormones activate and stimulate a sluggish adrenal, nurture and nourish this endocrine gland, and enable it to pour forth its valuable cortisone, the same hormone that is artificially administered to those with arthritic distress. An all-natural program that emphasizes intake of healthful hormone foods, may well be the key to obtaining natural cortisone through nourishment of the adrenal glands.

HOW GLANDULAR METABOLISM CORRECTION MAY PROMOTE NATURAL CORTISONE STIMULATION. It is generally recognized that arthritic-rheumatic distress has its beginning in an error in endocrine glandular metabolism. The adrenal glands, in particular, have become weak or sluggish, and their hormone supply becomes diminished. The cortex (outer portion) is a shell made up of cells which create hormones known as "steroid hormones." Of the more than 30 hormones that should be issued by a healthy and well-nourished cortex, one stands out as the key to glandular metabolism—*cortisone*. A deficiency of this hormone has been seen to be the basic cause of erroneous glandular metabolism as well as a variety of symptoms, foremost of which are those in the arthritic

52

group. Failure or decline of the cortex of the adrenal gland to supply its valuable hormones is seen as the basic root cause of arthritic distress. While synthetic cortisone has been administered to help make up for the deficiency, there is an increasing desire to aid the adrenal glands to become *naturally stimulated* so a natural supply of cortisone is issued to ease arthritic distress. By helping to correct this metabolic defect through glandular balance, hormones help establish a rhythmic "biological clock" to promote a feeling of well-being and relief from arthritic symptoms.

How a "Mineral Broth" Helps Relieve Arthritic Acidosis

An all-natural "Mineral Broth" hormone food reportedly helps correct problems of acidosis, a condition that interferes with hormone metabolism and is contrary to the healthy functioning of the cortisone-issuing adrenal glands. To help re-establish a healthful glandular balance, this Mineral Broth hormone food should be taken in the morning, every single day.

MINERAL BROTH. In a large stainless steel kettle, place the following: two potatoes, chopped or sliced; one cup diced carrots; one cup celery, leaves and all, chopped; one cup of any available vegetable tops, such as beet or turnip tops. Add one quart milk, cover, and cook moderately for 30 minutes. Strain off liquid, cool until warm, then drink. NOTE: To store, keep in refrigerator and warm up before serving.

How the Mineral Broth Helped Ease Adele's Early Morning Stiffness. Adele R. used to awaken all tied up in knots. The early morning hours were the worst for her stiff limbs. It took her up to an hour to "unwind" the kinks from her stiff arms and legs. She would often drink up to three cups of coffee, laced with sugar, accompanied by cake and canned fruit—all rich in refined sugar. Adele R. thought this would give her "energy," but it caused an imbalance in her calcium-phosphorus ratio, her glands became sluggish, and her hormone deficiency was a prime cause of her arthritic weakness. Now, she gave up the early morning coffee-sugar habit, and turned to the Mineral Broth hormone food.

Minerals Help Her Feel Joyful in the Morning. Adele R. benefited from the Mineral Broth (which was highly alkaline) because it helped to ease acidosis (a symptom of excessive caffeine-sugar intake) and nourished her adrenal glands. With a healthy hormone rhythm, she felt more flexible and joyful in the morning.

But a problem arose by noontime. She would fall back on her habitual imbibing of sugar-laced soda pop and lots of coffee, along with excessive eating of sugar and sweets. By early afternoon, she was again twisted up with gnarled muscles. She often complained that she felt "all tied up in knots." Yet, she could not give up her sweets compulsion and this interfered with promoting a healthful hormone rhythm. While the Mineral Broth hormone food offered hope for healing, it was just *one* natural law of healthful living. The other natural laws call for elimination of artificial sweets, starches, and synthetic foods.

The All-Natural Mineral Program to Restore Hormone Balance

In a reported program to help establish a natural mineral-hormone balance, there was much relief of arthritic unrest by assisting the adrenal glands, as well as other body glands, in becoming adequately nourished. Under this program, the adrenal glands are especially benefited by the high mineral nourishment, enabling the cortex to stimulate healthful cortisone production through all-natural means. This is the key to helping restore hormone balance and correcting metabolic defects, thereby easing arthritis distress.

1. *Eliminate Sugar.* All sugar-containing foods (these include bleached white bread and packaged products made from such devitalized flour) should be eliminated. *Benefit:* Sugar is highly acid; many arthritics experience discomfort by first developing problems of acidosis. Elimination of sugar foods helps ease the high supply of acid, often the forerunner of arthritis. The adrenal glands have to work swiftly to cooperate with the other glands to metabolize sugar. This causes an overworking of the glands and a general weakening. A deficiency of cortisone is the consequence of an exhausted glandular network. Help your adrenals issue cortisone by eliminating sugar so that your glands may work without interference from unnatural foods.

2. *Increase Intake of Fresh Fruits and Vegetables.* These natural hormone foods are prime sources of precious minerals needed to feed the adrenal glands. *Benefit:* Fresh fruit and vegetable minerals will help protein to form, influence glandular response, control hormones that send nutrients to millions of body cells and tissues, and prompt the adrenal glands to issue a healthful supply of arthritis-relieving natural cortisone.

3. *A Raw Juice Fast Helps Flush Out Corrosive Impurities.* Minerals in freshly squeezed, raw juices offer an alkaline surplus to balance the acids which are in large quantity in the blood and tissues, when the adrenal glands are malfunctioning. Go on a raw juice fast for an entire day. The benefit here is that fasting will cleanse the system (notably the glands) of accumulated impurities, enabling them to issue forth a sparkling, healthful supply of valuable hormones.

4. *Seed Oils Work with Minerals to Establish Hormone Rhythm.* Oils from safflower, sunflower, cottonseed, corn, wheat, and other seed-bearing plants are especially useful in helping to establish a hormone rhythm. These unsaturated fatty acids combine with minerals to create a molecular structure that works to improve body metabolism. The adrenal glands are thus soothed and refreshed, as well as nourished, by the intake of these seed oils. Use these oils in salads as well as in cooking as a butter substitute.

NATURAL HORMONE BOOSTER ELIXIR. Combine one-half glass apple juice, one-half glass seasonal berry juice, and four tablespoons of any cold-pressed seed oil. Stir vigorously or put under blender for a moment. This Natural Hormone Booster Elixir is a prime source of minerals and unsaturated fatty acids that combine together to help nourish all the glands, especially the adrenals. Drink this Natural Hormone Booster Elixir twice daily, while following the other basic laws—an all-natural program of healthful living, with elimination of unnatural and synthetic foods.

5. *Stimulate a Sluggish Gland with Briskly Cool Showers.* By tradition and the experiences of hundreds of centuries, the briskly cold and health-boosting shower is able to have an exceedingly beneficial effect on the entire body. An old-fashioned cold shower (it should be comfortable and not freezing cold!) will help boost circulation, pep up muscle tone and nerve force, and speed up metabolism. Once the metabolism has been boosted, the various glands, as well as the adrenals, will pick up their function and increase hormone production. A morning shower that is briskly cool is a good "gland exercise" that helps the adrenal cortex issue forth a much needed supply of cortisone.

Health Hints for Healthy Adrenal Glands: To help maintain healthy adrenal glands, it is advisable to eliminate any sharp condiments, such as salt, vinegar, mustard, ketchup, and pepper. Eliminate coffee, tea (except all-natural herbal teas), tobacco, and alcohol. Eliminate anything made with white sugar or white flour. Eliminate refined or processed foods which are almost always chemically saturated and treated with salts and harsh condiments. By eliminating these artificial non-foods, your adrenal glands will not need to work overtime in their harsh metabolism; the adrenals can then work upon wholesome and less-taxing, all-natural foods, and be able to issue forth a healthy supply of cortisone, needed to soothe arthritic aches and distress.

How to Feed Minerals to Your Glandular System and Ease Arthritic Unrest

Minerals in wholesome hormone foods will help detoxify the bacteria of infection, aid in metabolizing food, draw out nourishing substances from these foods, and help invigorate the adrenals. Minerals basically nourish these glands and stimulate them to secrete their valuable hormones. To feed minerals to your adrenals, here is a little guide to follow:

CALCIUM. Circulates in the soft body tissues and fluids and promotes regulation of liquid passage through the walls of the tissues and cells. Calcium helps ease problems of arthritic osteoporosis or brittle bones. The glands need to use this mineral in the manufacture of their hormones in order to ease arthritic distress. *Food Sources:* All dairy and milk products, natural cheese, green vegetables, kale, broccoli, collards.

PHOSPHORUS. The cells of the adrenal glands are rich in phosphorus. The adrenals use phosphorus to convert oxidative energy to cellular work, to help in the secretion of cortisone and some 30 other hormones. The adrenals also need this mineral to neutralize excess acidity (seen in many arthritics) and to keep a healthy alkaline balance. *Food Sources:* All dairy products, natural cheese, poultry, fish, peas, whole grain cereals, beans, nuts.

IRON. The adrenal tissues and cells need iron to provide them with oxygen. The adrenals then take this iron and use it as an energy media from which they make valuable hormones. The adrenals also use the iron to improve the health and color of your bloodstream. *Food Sources:* Liver, kidney, egg yolk, green leafy vegetables, dried fruits, molasses, cherries, raisins, grapes.

IODINE. This mineral is highly concentrated in the adrenal cortex. It is used to help send a stream of healthful nourishment to the cerebro-spinal fluid and nourish the body's skeletal structure. The hormones are rich in iodine and a deficiency may mean a reduction in the supply of needed cortisone. *Food Sources:* Salt-water seafood, sardines, eggs, oatmeal, potato with skin, cabbage, garlic.

SODIUM. The adrenal glands need *natural* sodium from foods to help issue its valuable arthritis-easing hormones. In particular, the adrenals use sodium to help influence the osmotic pressure and fluid passage between tissues and blood. The adrenal hormones deposit this *natural* sodium in the muscular and neuron system, easing stiffness and kinkiness. A special benefit is that the hormone sends this mineral into the bloodstream to help redissolve coagulated fibrin, a forerunner of stiff fingers and joints. *Food Sources:* Meats, fish, poultry, milk, natural cheese, beets, Swiss chard, beet greens, celery, carrots.

POTASSIUM. The adrenal glands join this mineral with sodium to help control body fluids and the metabolic processes. Potassium works upon the glands to help dispose of waste substances, a vital process in the cleansing of the arthritic's system. *Food Sources:* All citrus fruits, watercress, mint leaves, green peppers, alfalfa tea, sea plants such as kelp. NOTE: A powerhouse of potassium for your adrenal glands is that of *raw potato juice.* The high alkaline and potassium supply is a dynamic food for sluggish adrenals and may well be the "tonic" needed to boost a natural cortisone hormone flow.

MAGNESIUM. The adrenal glands use magnesium as a "starter" for the internal biochemical reactions to help boost the production of cortisone, among other hormones. Another benefit is that the adrenal glands use magnesium to help form blood albumen, which acts as a catalyst for assimilating carbohydrates so that the body will not be overloaded with fat. This is an internal metabolism that helps promote a rhythmic flow of harmonious hormones, unimpeded by excess fat. *Food Sources:* Whole grains, beans, dairy foods, egg yolks, coconut.

COPPER. The adrenal glands work to metabolize foods into hemoglobin by using copper. This mineral is food for the adrenals, which are able to transform ingested foods into the substances from which hormones are made. In particular, the adrenals need copper to help create oxidation of tyrosine, an amino acid that influences utilization of Vitamin C to help build and rebuild the tissues of the body and the components of the skeletal structure. It is this natural harmony that helps ease problems of formation of arthritis. *Food Sources:* Beef liver, calves' liver, almonds, apricots, black mission figs, loganberries, English walnuts, blackstrap molasses, egg yolk.

SULPHUR. The adrenal glands use sulphur to help invigorate the bloodstream and resist bacterial infections that are often found in the "bone pockets" where arthritis develops. The adrenals use sulphur to promote protein metabolism and send prepared amino acids into the hormones it issues. Cortisone, as it is manufactured by a mineral-nourished adrenal gland, contains a good amount of sulphur. *Food Sources:* Cabbage, molasses, Brussels sprouts, red currants, cranberries, pineapples, Brazil nuts, dried chestnuts.

SILICON. The adrenal glands take up silicon and use it to help build strong muscles, connective tissues, and feed the skin and cellular walls. Silicon is a part of the adrenal hormones which bestows a "knitting repair" benefit on brittle or sponge-like bone structures. It is often regarded as the "youth mineral" in hormones. *Food Sources:* Whole grain foods, lentils, mushrooms, liver, tomatoes, carrots, buckwheat. All foods made from natural buckwheat are rich in silicon, the youth mineral for the adrenal hormones.

ZINC. The adrenal glands, themselves, have a good supply of this mineral, which they use to help metabolize some proteins and carbohydrates to help keep the skeletal structure feeling resiliently youthful. Zinc, in the hormones, helps the body assimilate sugars and starches; it creates a valuable "joint flexibility" power by enabling the hormones from the adrenals to take in oxygen and expel carbon dioxide and toxic wastes. This forms an "internal scrubbing" that helps keep the limbs in a youthfully healthful condition. When the adrenals absorb zinc for their hormones, the "stream" works in carbohydrate utilization and this tends to create biological energy; the youthful resiliency of "young feeling" fingers and toes and joints may well depend upon this important adrenal food, zinc. *Food Sources:* Green leaves of vegetables, egg yolk, seeds, nuts, beans, peas.

Magic Hormone Foods Promote "Forever Young" Family of Glands. The complete set of minerals in hormone foods work closely together to help promote a feeling of youthfulness in the system, by nourishing the network of body glands, notably the adrenals. When these minerals "adjust" the "adrenal clock," they help promote a "time release action" of healthy hormones (cortisone is the forerunner), that works to ease arthritic unrest and bring about a feeling of youth in the body's joints.

A Simple Mineral-Feeding Program Relaxed John's Stiffening Joints. As a lathe operator, John C. needed flexible fingers and free-moving skeletal joints to manage his complicated machine in the sprawling factory. When he felt his muscles tied up "in knots" and an invisible pressure between his shoulder blades, he thought it was just due to prolonged hours of standing up. But when the tight muscles became like "gnarled fists" and he experienced a numbing sensation in his fingers and knees, he realized that he was not just tired, but that he had rheumatic-like symptoms.

Faulty Diet Clue to Glandular Unrest. Because John C. had to work long hours, he had no time for more healthful eating; he would usually eat cold meat sandwiches on white bread with sugar-laden coffee and processed, packaged cakes. This created less-than-healthy metabolism, as tests from the endocrinologist pointed out. He learned that the nutritionally deprived adrenal glands had diminished the rhythmic supply of valuable youth-giving cortisone. His other glands were similarly tossed out of kilter since the entire network of body glands work in an interconnected rhythm. If one is malfunctioning, the others are adversely influenced, as in a chain of connected links. When John C.'s mineral-undernourished adrenals slowed up the necessary production of its over 30 hormones, and a deficiency of cortisone led to his pain-wracked stiffening fingers and joints, he began to develop arthritic-like symptoms. This forced him to correct his living methods.

Simple Mineral-Eating Plan. Here is what John C. did in following a program to help restore the rhythmic action of the biological clock of the family of glands within his system:

1. *Brisk, Cool Shower in Morning.* John C. took a five-minute brisk, cool shower (needle sprays are especially invigorating to the glands) in the morning. This helped spark up the function of his glands and other body processes in the early morning, when they might normally be sluggish and "sleepy" after a night's rest.

2. *Fresh Berry Juice.* Before breakfast, a glass of fresh berry juice offered a treasure house of minerals and vitamins, as well as enzymes, that stoked the fires of his glandular furnace. The resultant "heat" was the rhythmic stream of hormones.

3. *Fruit Salad at Breakfast.* A fresh fruit salad at breakfast provided his system with a powerhouse of enzymes and other nutrients that sparked the minerals to enter into the endocrine gland process. Raw fruit is especially beneficial because it contains a nature-endowed source of those same minerals that are found in the hormones, themselves!

4. *Protein Food Provides Adrenal Activation.* A protein food at breakfast, such as egg, fish, meat, cheese, beans, and nuts, offered a

supply of essential amino acids that later proved to boost and activate the adrenal glands to issue their rhythmic hormone flow to help nourish the body's organs and provide impetus to its processes.

5. *Natural Beverages Are Soothing.* For a warm beverage at breakfast (the warmth is essential to the adrenal glands and digestive system, *at the end of a meal,* to help promote cortisone manufacture), John C. sipped a non-caffeine coffee substitute, a cup of herb tea, or a mixture of blackstrap molasses (two tablespoons) in a cup of boiled water. This is a powerhouse of minerals needed by the body's glands.

6. *Noontime Meals Were Raw Vegetables.* At noon, John C. would make time, despite the heavy schedule at his machine, to have a plate of raw vegetables mixed with a salad dressing of equal parts of lemon juice and apple cider vinegar, with one-half teaspoon of organic honey. This gave him a rich supply of vitamins, minerals, proteins, and enzymes, together with a good proportion of unsaturated fatty acids. His beverage was a coffee substitute or herb tea. This, again, offered him a natural source of nutrients. *Benefits:* At noontime, the glands began to feel the physical-mental pressure of work and required nourishment via all-natural sources. The raw vegetable meal offered an abundance of such nutrients. PROTEIN SUPPLEMENT: John C. might have a side dish of broiled liver or fat-trimmed meat slices.

7. *For His Evening Meal, He Ate High-Protein Foods for Hormone Invigoration.* The evening meal emphasized protein to help provide more amino acids for the glands. When the adrenals were fed sufficient protein, they issued forth an invigorated series of "hormone rivers" that provided nourishment to his so-called tired bones and joints. A high-protein source was meat, fish, poultry, soybeans, or cheese. Again, he would have a raw vegetable salad to provide minerals which worked to boost amino acid power to feed the adrenals and other glands.

8. *A Return to Nature Meant a Glandular Return to Youth.* John C. eliminated artificial sugar-starch-salt foods; he saw to it that he obtained at least eight hours of healthful sleep each night; he took frequent "rest breaks" and was careful about his eating programs. It took him close to three months before he was able to feel "young again" and be able to open and close his fingers with the flexibility of an adolescent! His back felt strong. His posture was erect. His skin and hair glowed with the radiant look of youth. He could walk and bend with youthful resiliency. His well-nourished glands had helped

put youth into his formerly arthritic-like fingers and muscles. It is hoped he will continue to follow this all-natural way of better health to help avoid the possibility of a recurrence of his prematurely aging rheumatic distress.

The All-Natural Hormone Food That Awakens Your Glands to Promote the Reward of "Young Feeling" Fingers and Muscles

European physicians report the success of an all-natural hormone food in helping to relieve and heal unnaturally stiff fingers and arthritic-like distress amongst their patients.

Brewer's Yeast Boosts "Young Feeling" Fingers. The all-natural food, Brewer's Yeast, is a rich source of a nutrient known as pantothenic acid—part of the complex molecule of co-enzymes which becomes concerned with the mineral-gland metabolism of proteins, fats, and carbohydrates. Together, pantothenic acid in Brewer's Yeast with mineral supplements, formed a natural cortisone flow, in conjunction with sterols and steroid hormones, which worked to promote a feeling of "young again" fingers and joints in patients treated by these European physicians.

Two Natural Hormone Foods Rejuvenate Joints. A team of researchers[1] noted that rheumatoid arthritics had unnaturally low blood pantothenic acid levels. The lower the level, the greater the severity of their arthritic distress. The doctors gave these arthritics a daily supply of two natural substances—organic honey and pantothenic acid, as found in Brewer's Yeast. These two natural foods combined and reportedly raised the pantothenic acid level in the bloodstream. *Benefits:* The two natural hormone foods stimulated the adrenal glands to issue a healthy supply of natural cortisone. The patients experienced a general improvement—a rejuvenation of the joints and mobility of formerly stiff fingers and limbs. In conjunction with other natural health programs, the daily use of organic honey and Brewer's Yeast provided this "rejuvenation." Truly, it's all in the glands! Feed the glands and rejuvenate your body!

Adrenals Improve with Daily Amounts of Brewer's Yeast. Several other patients[2] who had osteoarthritis were given daily amounts of Brewer's Yeast alone, to feed the adrenals the much-needed pantothenic acid. *Benefits:* There was considerable improvement in the

---

[1] *Lancet,* 2:862; Oct. 26, 1963.
[2] *Lancet,* 2:1168; Nov. 30, 1963.

stiff fingers. When the Brewer's Yeast was withdrawn from their diet, the patients experienced a return to stiff fingers and limbs.

HOW THIS HORMONE FOOD PROGRAM WILL HELP IM-PROVE GLAND POWER. This simple program calls for the daily and regular use of Brewer's Yeast (for the rich supply of pantothenic acid) and organic honey (for the rich mineral supply), which work together to feed the adrenals and other glands.

Boosts Cortisone Manufacture. The nutrients in this "Yeast Tonic," as it came to be known, fed the adrenals. They worked to help the adrenals secrete cortisone—particularly, desoxycortisone, or DOC. This cortisone hormone helped the body fight off arthritic infections by setting up a "shield" around bacteria and toxic substances, thus preventing them from spreading to surrounding tissues. (It's a "holding principle," much the same as that used in controlling a forest fire.)

Adrenal cortisone then summons blood and tissue fluids and white blood cells to come to the aid of the arthritic-like area. There may be some swelling and pain, and even fever, but the rest of the body is protected. The "fire" is controlled.

Cortisone Supply Must Be Available Through Yeast Tonic. The hormone cortisone holds the hormone DOC in check. But there must be a ready supply of adrenal-issued cortisone available. This is possible through the "Yeast Tonic" and other described natural hormone food health programs. NOTE: A deficiency of minerals and nutrients means a deficiency of cortisone. If this happens, then DOC runs rampant and the inflammation becomes like a ravaging forest fire, increasing yearly, leading to severe arthritis and premature rheumatic joint-limb stiffening. To enjoy "health insurance," it is essential to follow the simple, yet remarkably effective natural health hormone food program used by European doctors—the "Yeast Tonic" which helps provide the minerals needed by the adrenals to manufacture natural cortisone.

HOW TO MAKE YOUR OWN "YEAST TONIC." In one glass of tomato juice, place four heaping tablespoons of Brewer's Yeast powder or flakes (sold at health food stores or herbal pharmacies), then add two tablespoons of organic natural honey. Stir vigorously. For good results, put in blender and whirr for two minutes. Drink one glass of your "Yeast Tonic" every single morning. You will be sending a rich stream of vitamins, minerals, pantothenic acid, and enzymes into your glandular network, especially to your adrenals. The nutrients in the "Yeast Tonic" help send power to the adrenals, which then issue healthful cortisone that acts as a "guard" to control the DOC hormone until the latter can destroy its "imprisoned" infectious bacteria. This biological rhythm generated by hormone foods helps ease problems of arthritic-rheumatic disorder and helps keep the joints and limbs feeling smoothly resilient and young.

NATURAL "FEEL YOUNG" HORMONE TONIC. Two natural foods—celery juice and honey—can be prepared in a tonic to help invigorate the adrenal glands to issue forth a healthful supply of cortisone, needed to make your joints and limbs "feel young" again.

In a glass, mix celery juice with two tablespoons of organic honey. Drink daily. SPECIAL TIP: Add Brewer's Yeast to offer a booster. BENEFITS: Celery has an alkaline reaction, which is soothing to "burning joints." The honey and Brewer's Yeast offer a *combination* of minerals and pantothenic acid to help strengthen the power of the adrenals to issue forth the valuable cortisone.

The hormone food in this "Feel Young" Hormone Tonic helps correct sluggish metabolism and speeds up the biochemical processes to help promote tissue regeneration, protein synthesis, and antibody production—and, most important—it helps manufacture a natural cortisone to be distributed widely throughout the body, which firms up the muscles, loosens up stiff fingers and limbs, and, indeed, makes the person "feel young" with nature.

OTHER SOURCES OF PANTOTHENIC ACID. Natural food sources include liver, kidney, heart, salmon, and eggs. Mushrooms, broccoli, beef tongue, peanuts, and soybean flour are still more good sources. The dark meat of turkey has twice as much pantothenic acid as does the white meat. Organ meats are more important sources than muscle meats. Try lentils, sesame and sunflower seeds, brown rice, sardines, watermelon, and wild rice. MOST POTENT SOURCE: Brewer's Yeast has about 12 times as much as any other source, along with vitamins, minerals, enzymes, and amino acids—all of which work together to nourish the glandular network and the adrenals, and especially to issue valuable youth-building cortisone.

How Women Can "Rejuvenate" Through Mineral-Enriched Glands

Barbara J. was "doubled over" with such knife-like pains in her lower back, that she could scarcely sit up to do ordinary housework. Bending over to vacuum a rug meant it was a painful experience to try to straighten up again. She refused to believe the condition was arthritis because she had a hopeful outlook for the years ahead. She felt it was only a temporary backache that would go away. But her hopes were in vain. The pains increased.

Metabolism Correction Is Essential for Female Youthfulness. Her aging appearance prompted a relative to suggest a metabolism correction. The relative had been placed on a high calcium program. She explained that women are as susceptible as men because the hormonal changes in the early 40's induce depletion of the bone mineral content. It meant that Barbara's metabolism was in a negative balance because of the loss of minerals, and she might develop osteoporosis (a mineral depletion of the bones, leaving their normally solid structure pitted with sponge-like holes which consequently leaves them structurally weak and brittle). Barbara's bent-over pains were nature's warning symptoms that she had to correct her metabolism and boost her intake of hormone foods.

CALCIUM COCKTAIL. Barbara J. took four heaping tablespoons of powdered bone meal (sold at health stores and herbal pharmacies), which she mixed in a glass of whole milk or soybean milk. She would drink a glass of this "Calcium Cocktail" three times daily.

Benefits: The calcium helps balance two special hormones: the parathyroid hormone or PTH, which releases calcium from the bone into the blood, and thyrocalcitonin or TCT which prevents calcium loss. The minerals in the Calcium Cocktail lead to a prolonged suppression of parathyroid hormone function and a comparably enhanced stimulation of TCT secretion. *Results:* A restoration of a healthful calcium balance and improved storage of calcium, plus a better balance of calcium and phosphorus in the system to allow a more healthful absorption of both minerals. This helps maintain strong bones and muscular balance and promotes a feeling of youthful flexibility in the body's joints and limbs.

Barbara J. Is Able to Work and Twist with Youthful Agility. By helping to maintain this balance, Barbara J. was able to restore a healthful biological hormone rhythm and ease her symptoms. Soon, due to this hormone food, she could work and twist and bend with youthful agility. She takes the Calcium Cocktail three times daily. She follows other natural health programs and is able to correct the typical altered estrogen metabolism that often makes a woman so vulnerable to premature aging.

WHY WOMEN NEED MAGNESIUM TO PROMOTE YOUTHFUL FLEXIBILITY. Women, in particular, because of their middle-years hormonal changes, need one outstanding mineral—magnesium. This mineral keeps the pituitary gland from over-functioning, regulates her other body glands, and helps in producing hormones which "time release" the resorption of bone tissue into the blood. Magnesium feeds the pituitary so that the gland brings about a gradual and steady "nourishment" of the hormonal system. This helps ease problems of osteoporosis.

Magnesium helps re-establish normal balance, joining with other minerals to help ease symptoms of middle-years hormonal changes, thus nourishing the skeletal structure so it is youthfully flexible.

Food Sources of Magnesium: This mineral is found in dark green, leafy vegetables, soy flour (one of the richest sources), nuts, cashews, almonds, Brazil nuts, pumpkin seeds, and whole grains. NOTE: Cooking may deplete magnesium, so eat as many raw foods as possible.

Supplementary Sources of Magnesium. Health stores as well as herbal pharmacies have magnesium tablets. It is also found in an all-purpose, vitamin-mineral supplement capsule. Ocean plant foods such as kelp, dulse, algae, and seaweeds contain this mineral. A minimum intake of 500 milligrams of magnesium daily is healthful for women (and men, too) and could be a part of the all-natural program to help build youth through mineral-hormone-invigorated endocrine glands.

NOTE: The so-called arthritic-rheumatic disorder is *not* a single specific illness affecting only the joints. It exists in the organism as a whole, traced to a hormonic metabolic defect often caused by glandular imbalance. By following an all-natural program that includes natural hormone foods, special health tonics and better eating, moderate exercise, adequate nightly sleep, and elimination of synthetic and artificial foods, the adrenals and other glands can be sufficiently invigorated to become rejuvenated. The end result should be a healthful, re-established life rhythmic issuance of healthful cortisone and the other hormones so vital to happy and youthful living.

Summary

1. Improve youthful joint resiliency and flexibility by correcting glandular metabolism to promote natural cortisone stimulation.

2. A "Mineral Broth" eases arthritic acidosis and early morning stiffness.

3. Five simple all-natural steps help start restoration of hormone balance.

4. A "Natural Hormone Booster Elixir" energizes the adrenal glands.

5. Ten "Magic Minerals" in ordinary foods promote a "forever young" feeling in the family of body glands.

6. John C. nourished his adrenal glands and eased arthritic stiffness.

7. Brewer's Yeast and organic honey mixture became a "Yeast Tonic" that reportedly rejuvenated many European arthritic patients.

8. The Natural "Feel Young" Hormone Tonic boosts the natural cortisone stream.

9. Women are in special need of adrenal nourishment through a "Calcium Cocktail" and mineral-boosting program to help ease problems of middle-years stiffness.

10. Magnesium is believed to be the "youth mineral" that restores flexibility to the body's joints by activating the family of glands.

5

How Protein Breakfasts Help Promote Hormone-Energizing Youthfulness

A high-protein hormone food breakfast offers an early morning energizer to the glandular network, feeding and invigorating the sleepy pancreas, alerting it to a refreshing stimulation, so that the "biological clock" becomes adjusted to promote a steady hormone rhythm for most of the day's start. In particular, the hormones need this alerting in the morning to help perk up the body-mind combination and enable it to meet the responsibilities of the approaching day. It is in the high-protein breakfast foods you eat that you provide your glands with the hormone-feeding amino acids needed to perk up a healthful source of body-mind energy.

The Protein Breakfast Way to Hormone Rhythm. High-protein foods eaten at breakfast will alert the pancreas and the other glands to send forth a healthful and needed supply of hormones that work to establish a feeling of youthful vigor in the morning.

Here are the hormone benefits of a protein breakfast:

1. *Hormone Foods Enrich the Bloodstream.* Amino acids (metabolized protein) work to send a rich supply of hemoglobin to the bloodstream, creating a feeling of tingling warmth and vitality through blood hormones.

2. *Hormone Foods Strengthen Resistance to Infections.* The amino acids work to create antibodies which strengthen resistance against early morning sniffles, allergic unrest, and susceptibilities to sensitive contaminants.

3. *Hormone Foods Maintain Early Morning Body Water Balance.* A malnourished or underfed glandular system may cause a swelling of body tissues because of waterlogging. This is especially noticeable during the early morning hours. A high-protein breakfast sends a stream of amino-acid-sparked hormones to regulate the water balance of tissues and cells.

4. *Hormone Foods Prepare Cells and Tissues for the Day's Work.* In the form of amino acids, proteins spark the function of the body's glands to send forth hormones that work to help in the exchange of nutrients between cells and intercellular fluids, and between tissues and blood and lymph. NOTE: Morning or breakfast proteins are valuable in alerting sleepy glands to become healthfully awakened, so as to be able to send forth a "time release" or steady clock-rhythm hormonal supply, that provides a controlled and balanced amount of needed "youth-stream" energy and vitality.

5. *Hormone Foods Offer "Young Energy" Insurance.* In the form of amino acids, breakfast proteins are taken up by the pancreatic hormones and transformed into glucose and glycogen; in this form, they are stored in your liver to be doled out in a steady and rhythmic "clockwork" supply, providing you with youthful mind-body energy for most of the morning. Breakfast proteins become the source of this natural "young energy" insurance.

HEALTHY PROTEIN FOODS: Meats, fish, eggs, cheese, peas, beans, and nuts—these are the basic and all-important breakfast foods that are high in protein and essential vitamins, minerals, and enzymes, that are needed to alert the pancreas and other glands to send forth the rhythmic flow of hormones necessary to promote early morning and "foundation" energy for most of the waking hours of the day.

PROTEIN HORMONE FOOD EASES "LOW BLOOD SUGAR" TIREDNESS. A steady supply of protein in the early hours will help ease the problems of "low blood sugar" fatigue so often felt during the morning and even until noontime. Low blood sugar is known as hypoglycemia. This word is taken from two word derivatives—*hypo*, meaning below or lower than normal; *glycemia*, meaning sugar in the bloodstream. It is often the reverse of diabetes mellitus, in which there is an excess of sugar in the bloodstream due to inadequate utilization or secretion of the pancreatic hormone, insulin. Hypoglycemia causes a feeling of tiredness because insulin in the pancreas lacks the ingredients it normally uses to convey a feeling of alertness in the body. These ingredients are found in protein hormone foods. The amino acids are then taken up by insulin and sent to the other glands and body networks to help create a "chain reaction" of youthful vitality. Protein is seen to ease all-too-familiar early morning tiredness.

Protein Corrects Glandular Disorder. In low blood sugar or hypoglycemia, the pancreas (the gland located behind the lower part of the stomach) has become over-sensitive or over-active and produces too much insulin, instead of a normal amount. This is often noted when the person has eaten too much sweets and/or carbohydrates, and has become nervous because of a protein deficiency. This causes the stored up body sugar (or glucose) to be burned up rapidly. Protein offers a unique "hormone sparing" asset in that it works to promote a steady and soothing metabolization, so that the glands are able to function smoothly rather than erratically. NOTE: The brain cells depend wholly upon blood sugar or glucose for nourishment; deprived of this food, it may lead to mental sluggishness and a feeling of chronic fatigue. To help correct this problem, a high-protein breakfast offers a steady and rhythmic hormonal supply that self-regulates the internal source of glucose.

SIMPLE CORRECTION OF MALFUNCTIONING GLAND NETWORK. To help correct this pancreatic malfunctioning, the food program needs to be adjusted. Basically, the breakdown of the pancreas gland and the erratic or spasmodic flow of hormones is often brought on by over-stimulation of the islands of Langerhans (cells in the pancreas) by the excessive use of sweets, quickly absorbed starches, coffee, tobacco, alcohol, and soft drinks. By eliminating these non-foods, and substituting with a high-protein diet at breakfast time, there is hope for correction of this malfunctioning and an opportunity to promote a hormone-fed physical and mental alertness.

TEEN-AGE BOY RECOVERS FROM MORNING FATIGUE WITH HIGH-PROTEIN BREAKFAST. In one reported situation, teen-ager Robert E. was the victim of respiratory infections, asthmatic attacks that were more pronounced in the morning, and a feeling of chronic fatigue. Robert E. had tried a variety of treatments but they were only temporary. His mother was told about regulating his "hormone rhythm" through adjustment of his "gland clocks" with a high-protein breakfast. Here is the program she prepared for Robert E., after consulting with specialists:

1. In the morning, he was given a large glass of freshly squeezed fruit juice to provide his pancreas and other glands with needed and all-natural fruit sugar. *Added Benefit:* Large amounts of Vitamin C saturated the tissues and cells of the body's glands, strengthening them to function healthfully.

2. Robert E. was given a combination food supplement of Vitamin C (3,000 milligrams daily) and calcium (500 milligrams) in order to help provide even more cell food, as well as mineral food, for the pancreas.

3. Breakfast emphasized high-protein hormone foods, with low sugar and moderate carbohydrates.

Results: Reportedly, young Robert E. was able to control his asthmatic attacks, his mental-physical sluggishness eased, and he was soon alert and vigorous as a youngster should be. Now he follows a completely well-rounded hormone food nutritional regime.

Robert E. was prematurely aged because of this glandular weakness, and it illustrates that hormonal irregularities can strike anyone at any age, even in the youthful prime of life. However, with the adoption of a small food correction program, hope for "forever young" glands is provided for all ages.

Hormone Foods for Breakfast That Boost Morning "Gland Power"

Reportedly, healthful "gland foods" for breakfast include these:

Fruits: apples, apricots, berries, grapefruit, pears, melons, oranges, peaches, pineapples. These may be eaten raw or cooked, with or without cream. *NOTE:* Do not use sugar! If you purchase canned fruits they should be packed in water, not syrup. Read the label.

Vegetables: Asparagus, avocado, beets, broccoli, Brussels sprouts, cabbage, cauliflower, carrots, celery, cucumbers, corn, eggplant, lima beans, onions, peas, radishes, sauerkraut, squash, string beans, tomatoes, turnips, lettuce, mushrooms.

Beverages: Weak tea (tea ball, not brewed); decaffeinated coffee and coffee substitutes. Herb teas are advisable since they are free of caffeine and tannic acid. You may have club soda or dry ginger ale.

Main Foods: Meat, fish, eggs, non-processed cheeses, peas, beans, nuts.

AVOID THESE ANTI-GLAND FOODS: Spaghetti, macaroni, noodles, high-sugar and high-carbohydrate foods, pretzels, biscuits, wines, cordials, cocktails, beer, liquors, processed snacks, processed foods that have been made with sugar. The emphasis is upon *natural* foods, wholesome "high protein," and natural fruits and vegetables.

SAMPLE BREAKFAST: On arising, have an orange, one-half grapefruit, or a glass of freshly prepared fruit juice. For breakfast, have some more fruit or fruit juice, one egg with or without two slices of fat-trimmed meat, and one slice of whole grain bread with butter and a beverage.

The Two-Week "Breakfast Protein" Hormone Food Program to Help Boost Hormone-Energizing Powers

In a reported plan, a simple corrective food program helps introduce a steady and rhythmic supply of protein-energized hormones into the body, thereby promoting a healthy alertness in the early morning which is the foundation for the day. This program is offered as a general guideline to help boost natural sugar and healthful protein in the glandular network:

On Arising: Medium orange, four ounces of juice, or one-half grapefruit.

Breakfast: Fruit or four ounces of juice; one egg and one slice only of whole grain bread with butter; beverage.

Two Hours After Breakfast: Four ounces of juice.

Lunch: Fish, cheese, meat, or eggs; salad—large serving of lettuce, tomato, or apple salad with health store mayonnaise or health store French Dressing; vegetables, if desired. One slice of whole grain bread or toast, dessert, and beverage.

Three Hours After Lunch: Four ounces of milk.

Dinner: Soup, if desired (not thickened); vegetable; liberal portion of meat, fish, or poultry; one slice of whole grain bread; dessert and beverage.

Two-Three Hours After Dinner: Four ounces of milk.

Every Two Hours Until Bedtime: Four ounces of milk or a small handful of nuts.

BENEFITS: This reported program helps to readjust the malfunctioning "glandular clocks" and produces a *steady time-release hor-*

mone supply, which is used to regulate the steady, rhythmic glucose metabolism that produces a healthful and youthful mind-body energy in the early morning.

Special Benefit: The program offers a foundation of protein hormone food for the glands right in the early morning, when they need to be adjusted for the day's activities ahead. The entire day is influenced by the foods eaten at breakfast time! The above program and the emphasis on "high protein" for breakfast is the foundation for producing youthful hormones for most of the day.

Note: Many symptoms of premature fatigue and tiredness are felt in early mid-morning and mid-afternoon. For this reason, a hearty breakfast and between-meal feedings of mineral-rich milk or fruit are advised to prevent any slackening off of hormone-energized blood sugar levels which may occur some three hours after breakfast. Replace a coffee break with a "juice break" and experience a healthful hormonal lift that promotes the look and feel of youthful vitality!

How a Protein Hormone Food Breakfast Made Mike E. "Feel Young All Over"!

As a truckdriver, Mike E. had to awaken early and be on the road for a long drive to the other side of the state. His problem was that in the wee hours of the morning, his appetite was poor, his reflexes were slow (a symptom of a sluggish glandular function), and he was unable to keep wholesome food down.

It was easy to fall into the habitual pattern of drinking sugar-laced coffee and munching on pastries or sugary doughnuts and then taking off behind the wheel. Often Mike E. would bring along a thermos of sweetened coffee and a bag with a number of jelly doughnuts, sweet cakes, a hunk of cherry pie, or other confections. He would imbibe these sugary non-foods while on the road, in an effort to awaken his sluggish reflexes and boost his energy.

Mike E. soon found his senses becoming dulled, while his reflexes were all gnarled up. He made the wrong road turns, felt chronically irritated, and was completely disoriented. His vision was blurred. His hearing faculties were less than normal.

A near crash was responsible for alerting his supervisors to the need for giving Mike E. a complete physical examination. He had nearly gone off the road to avoid striking a car that was a comfortable distance away from him. But his nervous temperament was such that he envisioned the car attempting to drive right into his truck! It was time for a look-see into the causes for his erratic behavior.

The examination confirmed that his glandular responses were so awry because of the excessive sugar-sweet-caffeine intake, that his pancreas was disrupted and thrown into an upheaval. Further tests and discussions revealed that Mike E. ate more sweets and starches during noon, and this further tormented his pancreas and the network of related glands. This improper diet caused a malfunctioning of the biological gland clocks and the hormone rhythm was disrupted.

SIMPLE, YET EFFECTIVE HORMONE-BOOSTING BREAKFAST PLAN. Mike E. was told to eat a breakfast consisting of a soft-boiled egg, a bowl of fresh fruit, one slice of whole grain bread with butter pat (optional was a slice of broiled meat), and a cup of coffee substitute.

Benefits: The high protein in the above foods was taken by the metabolic system and broken down into amino acids which alerted a sluggish pancreas to issue forth a steady supply of its hormone, insulin, needed for assimilation in the system. The protein further nourished the pancreas and other glands to enable them to issue a "rhythmic hormonal" supply to keep Mike E. feeling alert and reasonably youthful (he was 38, yet felt double that age because of poor hormone nourishment), and this enabled him to become a safe driver and worker.

Then a problem ensued that caused him to lose his job. He might have had a nourishing breakfast, but at noontime he would again imbibe coffee laced with sugar and eat excessively heavy carbohydrate foods so that his impulses were erratic and his hormone supplies became spasmodic. Another near accident cost him his job. It is sad because he had openly explained, after the natural protein breakfast was followed for two weeks, that it made him "feel young all over."

BANANA-CEREAL-MILK BREAKFAST OFFERS "INSTANT NOURISHMENT" FOR THE GLANDS. Three natural hormone foods offer a treasure of nutrients that work speedily to alert and arouse the glands at a time in the morning when they are yearning for invigoration. In combination, they offer the ingredients sought by the glands so they can create a rhythm of youthful hormones within the body. Here are the three natural hormone foods and their hormone benefits:

1. *Banana.* The natural fruit sugars of the banana are reported to be from 96.0 to 99.5 per cent utilizable, highly digestible, and also protein-sparing when taken up by the gland network. This hormone-producing benefit is maximally effective when protein and fruit sugars are ingested simultaneously. Therefore, in the morning, a banana eaten with a protein food, offers a well-balanced and time-release benefit to the gland system, enabling it to issue forth an equally well-balanced rhythm of hormone lifestreams. SPECIAL TIP: The fruit sugars of the banana are especially high and utilizable in very ripe bananas. Fully ripened fruit is preferable. If you have green bananas, let them ripen at room temperature before eating, in order to benefit from the rich supply of natural hormone-feeding fruit sugars.

2. *Cereal.* Your glands require the protein and natural carbohydrates of "whole grain," non-processed cereals. These are available in most health food stores as well as special diet shops. Whole grain cereals offer carbohydrates that work speedily to alert the pancreas and related endocrines; they also maintain the blood sugar at a steady hormone-producing level. These cereal carbohydrates regulate body water metabolism, ease the hunger sensation, and help promote a hormone-washed feeling of comfortable satisfaction. Proteins in the whole grains work to help the pancreas maintain a steady blood sugar, send forth healthy hormones that improve instinctive reactions, boost the neuromuscular network, boost strength and endurance, and improve the supply of oxygen required to perform a specified amount of work. In *combination,* the carbohydrates, proteins, and vitamins-minerals in whole grain cereals work to adjust the biological gland clocks and improve the mind-body responses in the morning.

If you prefer, make your own power-packed hormone-feeding breakfast cereals with these two time-tested traditional recipes:

Millet Cereal. One-half cup hulled millet, one cup water, one cup milk, one tablespoon honey.

Bring water and milk to boil in top part of double boiler. Add millet. Boil five minutes, then steam over boiling water for 30 minutes. Add honey (raisins, dried fruit) and steam five minutes longer. *Serves 4-6.*

This Millet Cereal offers a natural source of grain carbohydrates as well as protein and minerals that work in harmony to adjust the biological gland clocks in the early morning, helping to create a healthful rhythm of hormone lifestreams. The *unique benefit* is that the whole grain Millet Cereal breakfast food offers an *alkaline* source as well as nutrient power. Protein-minerals-enzymes-carbohydrates work more favorably upon the glands when treated to this alkaline environment.

Five-Minute Hormone Food Breakfast Booster. In one pan, place one tablespoon whole wheat flour, two tablespoons whole wheat bran, two tablespoons whole flaxseed, two chopped figs or soaked prunes. Cover with water. Boil just five minutes. Stir briefly to prevent scorching. Serve promptly with a bit of organic honey or whole milk. *Serves 1-2.*

This Five-Minute Hormone Food Breakfast Booster is a prime source of grain carbohydrates and an especially potent source of natural fruit sugars and protein, with good amounts of minerals. Together, all the nutrients work to alert the glands and boost the ability of the pancreas to draw upon a slow and rhythmic supply of stored glycogen to provide a hormone rhythm that creates youthful energy in the morning. The *special benefit* of the Five-Minute Breakfast Booster is that its combination of nutrients work to promote glandular utilization of nitrogen, calcium, phosphorus, and iron so that the hormone is of an especially youthfully rich quality, providing a clear mind and a youthfully resilient body.

3. *Milk.* Whole milk, preferably from cows who graze on organic soil, is a magnificent source of what is known as dynamic protein, which is a rich source of those amino acids needed to invigorate and stimulate the entire early morning glandular network to promote a healthful supply of energizing hormones. Milk combines with the other foods to promote better utilization of hormone-making nitrogen, calcium, phosphorus, iron, thiamine, and niacin. Milk helps *retain* these nutrients and establishes a healthful balance, needed by the endocrine network for manufacture of energy-youth-building hormones in the morning: the foundation for the rest of the day!

A combination of banana, natural cereal, and whole milk, therefore, can be considered as the spark plug that helps set off the rhythm and motion of the hormone-gushing endocrine glands, to promote vital energy in the early morning hours.

ON-THE-ROAD MORNING TONIC. For those who have to travel, cannot eat immediately upon arriving, or absolutely refuse to eat breakfast, a time-tested, On-the-Road Morning Tonic may be taken about an hour after leaving home.

How to Make It: Mash one fully ripe banana in a container of cool milk. Drink slowly. Use a spoon to scrape out the banana.

The benefit of the On-the-Road Morning Tonic is that it will help stimulate the glandular network so that there is a sufficient awakening of the sluggish hormone-producing pancreas. It is usually a palatable and naturally sweet "breakfast food" for the most stubborn of morning appetites. The fine, fibrous cellular material works to promote digestive satisfaction and an internal cleansing, all at the same time.

WHOLE GRAIN CEREALS REJUVENATE GLAND RESPONSES. Breakfast with whole grain cereals helps improve and rejuvenate the response reflexes of the glandular system. Whole grain cereals, with their bran, germ, and endosperm are rich in the concentrated sources of "gland food," such as protein, the B-complex vitamins, iron, and phosphorus; particularly, two amino acids—*lysine* and *tryptophane*—are powerhouses of gland nourishment. Both of these amino acids work to help alert the pancreas to reconstitute the B-complex vitamins into ingredients found in the hormones, themselves, and to improve the powers of a sluggish early morning metabolism. These two amino acids are the keys to rejuvenation of the glandular system and the promotion of a healthful rhythm of youthful hormones.

Hormone-Boosting Whole Grain Foods

Help the rhythm of the endocrine gland hormones with any of these whole grain foods:

Buckwheat Flour—the finely ground product obtained by sifting buckwheat meal, rich in vitamins, minerals, and protein.

Oatmeal—also called rolled oats, and a prime source of nutrients needed to regulate normal and healthful blood sugar in the early morning hours.

Soy Products—regarded as close to animal protein and rich in nearly all known amino acids, which help awaken a sluggish pancreas and boost the rhythmic flow of valuable youth-building hormones. Obtain cold-pressed or cold-treated soy products, if possible, for a higher nutritional store.

Non-Processed Cereals Are Health-Plus for Glands. For a power-booster at breakfast time, select non-processed cereals. These retain the natural proportions of bran, germ, and endosperm, *and the specific nutrients that are part of the hormones, themselves!*

To help alert your early morning gland function, a healthful hormone food breakfast that is rich in proteins, is most beneficial. It offers a moderate low-fat, high-protein energy source for the glands, enabling them to "wake up" and provide you with a healthfully stimulating source of "feel young" hormones.

Summary

1. A protein breakfast helps awaken sluggish glands and promotes a "feel young" hormone rhythm.

2. A protein breakfast offers five distinctive hormone-boosting benefits.

3. Protein helps ease "low blood sugar" tiredness traced to a sluggish gland condition.

4. A simple improvement in breakfast helped Robert E. recover from respiratory problems and premature aging, by aiding his body in regulating "hormone rhythm" through natural means.

5. Special breakfast foods, available at most local food outlets, are able to boost morning "gland power."

6. Follow the two-week "Breakfast Protein" Program to help boost hormone-energizing powers.

7. Mike E. enjoyed "time-release hormone rhythm" by means of a simple improvement in his breakfast fare.

8. A Banana-Cereal-Milk Breakfast offers "instant nourishment" for the glands.

9. Treat your glands to a "forever young" hormone invigoration with the all-natural breakfast cereal recipes that boost metabolism and promote youthful energy.

10. Whole grain cereals often contain those very same substances that are found in hormones, themselves.

6

How Natural "Hormone Tonics" Help Create a "Think Young" Brain Power

Natural energizers in plant and seed juices reportedly have the ability to stimulate and nourish the pituitary-adrenal gland clocks, alerting them to issue forth a healthful rhythm of hormones that help create a youthfully invigorated brain power. These same energizers, when prepared in the form of health tonics and unique elixirs, are doubly effective because they are speedily absorbed by the glands, which then feel healthfully alerted to manufacture those hormones that work to stimulate the mental thinking processes. For many people, hormone tonics are as helpful as "brain foods."

How to Use Plant and Seed Juices to Improve Hormone-Boosted Brain Power

The natural raw juices from plants and seeds are prime sources of those substances which are needed by the pituitary gland to send a stream of rhythmically balanced hormones to the brain, which is used for boosting a youthful set of the essential five senses, as well as for helping stimulate sluggish thinking-memory processes.

Here's how to use this natural source of "brain food" with plant and seed juices:

1. *Fruit or Vegetable Juices Are Taken Up by the Pituitary as Food for the Brain.* In the process of metabolism, the pituitary gland

(the master controller of the body, located at the base of the brain) takes up the plant juices and uses its own "pigment" of carbon, hydrogen, oxygen, nitrogen, and iron, as well as vitamins-minerals-enzymes-amino acids, to help manufacture *at least 12 different hormones.* The nutrients in plant juices adjust the pituitary so it "ticks away" in clock form, sopping up these nutrients, which are used to spark the vital brain-feeding 12 hormones. These hormones then pep up the action of the two distinct parts of the pituitary, called the *lobes;* that is, the anterior and posterior parts, which need the hormones as activators to help stimulate the millions of brain cells which are part of the entire rhythm.

A unique benefit of plant juices is that the nutrients contain fruit sugar or fructose (also known as levulose). The hormones take this natural energy sugar and send it speedily streaming into the bloodstream, where it absorbs oxygen, which then goes streaming toward the brain. The tissues and cells of the brain require oxygen for "breathing." An oxygen deficiency may lead to brain suffocation or the so-called symptoms of premature senility. But fruit sugar and amino acids found in plant juices, when consumed together, will work in harmony to send a valuable stream of hormone-boosted oxygen to the brain to help stimulate healthfully normal thinking processes.

A pituitary gland that becomes adequately nourished by the fructose and amino acids in plant juices will speed up cellular processes and transform, expend, and convert that basic energy into a healthful, youthful, and vitalistic brain power!

2. *Seed Juices Help Adjust Rhythmic Hormone Balance to Improve Mental Stimulation.* The variety of available seed juices—or seed oils—offer hope for helping the pituitary create a rhythmic hormonal balance of steady hormones needed to nourish the brain and improve mental stimulation. Seed juices or oils, available in the form of wheat germ oil, sunflower seed oil, corn oil, avocado oil, almond oil, olive oil, linseed oil, peanut oil, soy oil, rice bran oil, and cottonseed oil, become lubricants for the "pituitary clock."

These lubricants work to help the pituitary send forth its rhythmic supply of over a dozen hormones that have this unique brain-boosting benefit:

Seed oils play a beneficial role in preventing oxygen from combining with essential fatty acids to form peroxides and substances known as "free radicals," which "coat" the cellular membranes of the brain and impede hormonal penetration and nourishment.

Nutrients in seed oils invigorate the pituitary gland to work in rhythmic harmony with the adrenals to send forth hormones that control cellular clogging and destruction, thereby maintaining metabolic balance. This helps maintain a supply of sufficient oxygen needed by the hormones to be transmitted via the bloodstream to the millions of brain cells as nourishment. Seed oils are regarded as anti-oxidants in that they nourish and stimulate the pituitary-adrenal combination to issue hormones that create internal rhythm and a healthful flow of oxygen—food for the brain!

Six "Think Young" Benefits of Natural Hormone Tonics

Metabolized juices from hormone foods such as fruits, vegetables, seeds, or grains, perform these six basic "think young" benefits via an alerted and invigorated pituitary-adrenal glandular rhythm:

1. *Steady Nerve Tension.* The juices and tonics help you maintain a youthful nerve response and promote relaxation from oxygen-starved, brain-induced tension.

2. *Help Improve the Basic Senses.* A rhythmic hormone flow to the brain will help improve the basic senses of sight, sound, hearing, smell, and touch. A nourished adrenal gland will issue its *cortin* hormone, which is secreted by the cortex (outer layer) and helps rejuvenate your basic five senses. A sluggish cortin supply will reduce the efficiency of these five basic senses.

3. *Boost Youthful Initiative.* An oxygen-nourished brain peps up the thinking processes and causes a feeling of alert youthfulness, which is needed to help improve initiative.

4. *Improve Desire for Work and Play.* Seed juices, in particular, alert the glands to manufacture hemoglobin, the vehicle by which brain-feeding oxygen is transported to its body cells and tissues; the brain is thusly oxygenated through the hemoglobin-carrying "breath of youth," and this creates a healthful and youthful desire to do normal work and engage in normal play.

5. *Improve Incentive in Living.* Juices help reset the biological gland clock so that the stream of hormones help liquefy arterial-like cholesterol plaques, which are the forerunners of premature aging and a decline in the normal incentive for healthful living. Juices help balance a rhythmical hormone flow through stimulation of the sluggish pituitary-adrenal network to help wash out the insides through a "hormone rejuvenation" and promote a healthful incentive for daily living.

6. *Prolong Healthful Youthfulness.* The set of rhythmic hormones work not only to nourish the brain, but also to help metabolize food more quickly into youthful energy, boost muscular power, and help build resistance to fatigue. In particular, plant juices offer speedily assimilating enzymes, fructose, and amino acids, which create natural hormone rivers to boost mental and physical endurance and help bring about a feeling of a "forever young" mind in a "feel young" body.

The "Hormone Tonics" That Helped Rose C. "Think Young"

Rose C. had frequent memory lapses. She was the nervous, worrying type who would fidget constantly. There were times when she would forget what items she wanted to purchase, after she had arrived at the store without having previously made a written list. At other times, she would display slow responses. Family and friends had to ask her the same question over and over again. When Rose C. finally replied, it was a vague, mumbling, incoherent response. She displayed symptoms of senility, although there were times when she seemed reasonably alert and responsive.

Well-meaning friends sought to save Rose C. from any institutional confinement since, in all other respects, she seemed pleasant and agreeable. But the problem was that she would swerve from one extreme of being very cooperative to the other extreme of being "edgy," nervous, and unable to think and act coherently.

This imbalance suggested a possible "hormone dysrhythm" that could be traced to "gland maladjustment."

Corrective Program to Adjust Gland Clocks. Several close members of the family sought to help correct Rose's life style and aid her body to become more nourished so it would be able to adjust its gland clocks and re-establish a healthful hormone rhythm. Here is the program they set up for Rose:

• Elimination of processed foods and all those containing artificial sugars, spices, synthetic flavorings, and additives.

• Emphasis upon a program of freshly squeezed fruit and vegetable juices to be sipped slowly throughout the day.

• Seed oils or plant juices were to replace all hard fats or saturated fats used for cooking and salads.

• One day per week was to be devoted to a raw juice fasting program, so that the ingredients in the juices could help lubricate the pituitary-adrenal and other glands and enable them to send oxygen-bearing hemoglobin to the brain to spark youthful responses and improve thinking-memory processes.

Here are some of the special "hormone tonics" that helped Rose C. "think young" again:

BRAIN DRINK. In a blender, mix one cup fresh or raw non-sweetened pineapple juice. Add one-half cup of any green leaves, whether in the form of lettuce, cabbage, organic tree leaves, watercress, parsley, chives, etc. Whirr quickly until thoroughly assimilated. Drink in the early morning. *Special Hormone Benefit:* The pineapple juice is a prime source of non-fermented enzymes which spark the blood pigment and solar energy of the green leaves to release the supply of easily assimilated vitamins-minerals-amino acids directly into the bloodstream. In combination, these nutrients from the Brain Drink work speedily upon the basic body glands, notably the pituitary and adrenals, to perform this vital function—to stimulate the bone marrow to produce hemoglobin, which is then energized by the hormones to go streaming to the brain to deposit valuable oxygen to the millions of brain tissues and cells. In the morning, when metabolic processes are slow, the Brain Drink can work quickly and without interference; hence, its unique benefit at the start of the day.

HORMONE TONIC. To help improve the quality of the hormones, themselves, take four tablespoons of any cold-pressed seed oil, mix in a glass of freshly prepared vegetable juice. Sprinkle with iodine-rich kelp or sea salt (iodine is needed by the thyroid as a hormone-boosting food). Drink this "hormone tonic" at noontime as well as in the late afternoon. *Special Hormone Benefit:* The treasure of minerals join with the unsaturated fatty acids and Vitamin E in the seed oil to promote more of a biological rhythm in the pituitary-adrenals and other glands. This causes a steady, "tick tock," clockwork, precision-like flow of hormones that serve to nourish the brain cells and help promote the youthful feeling that comes from well-lubricated and smoothly functioning body glands. The raw amino acids of the "hormone tonic" enter into the complex manufacture of constituents that are absorbed into the hormones, themselves, and then work to nourish and invigorate the "forever young" feeling of mind and body.

Rose C. Feels "Young in Mind" Again. It took close to three months of a return to an all-natural hormone food program and the daily nourishment of the gland foods through the tonics before Rose C. felt "young in mind" again. When the tonics nourished her pituitary-adrenal network, her thinking processes were revitalized, her well-oxygenated brain cells could perform smoothly, her memory was boosted, and she no longer forgot why she came to the store. In fact, she now felt so youthfully alert, she did not even need to prepare a shopping list! Her thinking and memory processes were hormone-invigorated with the instant responses of youth.

How Brain-Feeding Health Drinks Made a Salesman "Grow Younger"

As a traveling salesman, Oscar C. found it difficult to maintain regular or healthful living practices. His sleeping was irregular. Often he was up until the very late hours of the night, seeking out a potential sales client. At other times, he was on the road when he should have been in a comfortable bed. Mealtimes were also sporadic. He had to subsist on bleached, devitalized, pre-cooked, pre-packaged types of foods that had little or no nutritional value and offered a quick energy spurt that just as quickly subsided to produce chronic fatigue of mind and body.

Oscar C. did not feel his senses slipping all at once. There was a gradual numbing of his thinking processes. He would forget to mark down salient order points. He would take the wrong notations. He would fail to make certain routine appointment calls. As his condition worsened, he felt "mentally sluggish" and lost the desire to pursue what had always been his first love—selling! He thought he was getting old—at a little over 40! His incentives were lowered and he plodded along, each day resembling a heavy treadmill. He felt tired and "old."

THE BRAIN-NOG THAT HELPED REVERSE THE AGING PROCESS. It was while lunching with a client that he was treated to a special Brain-Nog, which the client said was a powerhouse of energy. The client explained that he always began the day with the Brain-Nog, and would even take some with him for lunch or for a "juice break," which he said would help him think better and feel more youthful "all over." The client invited Oscar C. to join him in a Brain-Nog.

Just one tall glass of a freshly prepared Brain-Nog served to sweep away the cobwebs, dusted out the pockets of Oscar's oxygen-starved brain cells, and helped him enjoy the benefits of a clear mind! He was amazed at the transformation. He actually felt young again, and he began to believe that the aging process had been reversed. Here is the special, easy-to-make Brain-Nog:

    1/2 cup chilled apricot juice
    1 teaspoon lemon juice
    Pinch of sea salt or kelp
    1 egg
    1½ cups milk

Shake well in a cocktail shaker or put in a blender; whirr for a moment or longer. Drink slowly.

Special Hormone Benefit of Brain-Nog: The iron in the apricot juice combines with the complete family of amino acids in the egg, to become "bound" by the Vitamin C of the lemon juice, and then be gathered up by the nutrients in the milk. The group of nutrients all work together to promote what is known as *coordination of hormonal activity.* The "binding" characteristic of these accumulated nutrients nourish the nerve fibers of the pituitary-adrenal system, enabling them to secrete a healthful and—most important—rhythmic clockwork beat of essential hormones. These hormones then absorb the iron, nourish the bone marrow, and take out the hemoglobin that becomes united with oxygen to feed the "starved" brain. The unique benefit of the Brain-Nog is that the aforelisted ingredients harmonize to send the valuable substances needed by the glands—in a healthful *combination*—to help create hormone *rhythm,* so that the brain and its related thinking processes will be sufficiently nourished to create sharp thinking actions, alert responses, and a "grow younger" feeling of body and mind.

How Seed Milk Helps Strengthen "Young Hormones"

An allergy to cow's or dairy milk made Lillian I. turn to seed milk. Lillian I. was seemingly healthy, except that there were times when her mind would wander, her thoughts became jumbled, and her fingers would not obey her impulses as speedily as they once did. When she began to break out in a skin rash because of cow's milk, she turned to seed milk. In this unexpected manner, she was able to so rejuvenate her glandular network, that her somewhat erratic mental weakness and sporadic emotional upheavals became corrected.

The glandular adjustment was undoubtedly due to the protein

power in seed milk, rather than her elimination of cow's milk, but it was a fortunate hint of nature that she make this change.

Here is how Lillian I. made:

Seed Milk Supreme for "Young Hormones"

1 cup seeds (sunflower, safflower, sesame, anise, carob, caraway, flaxseed, fennel, okra, etc.—use singly or in combination, according to taste)
1 cup cool water
2 tablespoons organic honey
Sprinkle of sea salt or dulse

Blend together well in an electric blender. Buzz until thoroughly mixed. Drink slowly—or serve over fruit, or use as the liquid in a cereal which contains whole grain products.

Special Benefits of Seed Milk Supreme for "Young Hormones": The milk drink is rich in valuable unsaturated fatty acids that join with the vitamins-minerals-protein and valuable enzymes to supercharge the pituitary and the other body glands, enabling them to manufacture a rich supply of hitherto sluggish hormones. It is this rich flow of rhythmic hormones that produces the "young feeling" of mind and body. *Special Unique Benefit:* The seed milk drink is a rich supply of those constituents from which the hormones, themselves, are made. The seed milk may well be regarded as "nature's hormones" in a healthful tonic. The seed milk has almost all of the essential amino acids needed to invigorate the hormones and enrich them with the magnetic power that triggers off the normal brain responses. This may well be the secret clue for its effectiveness in helping to create "young hormones" and a younger emotional state.

Follow Basic Health Rules. In addition to this Seed Milk Supreme for "young hormones," Lillian I. selected wholesome foods and eliminated all items made with or containing white sugar, white flour, artificial additives, and chemical colors. She would eat whole grain bread, fat-trimmed meats, poultry, fresh fish, and lots of raw vegetables, as well as plenty of raw fruit. She obtained sufficient nightly rest. Particularly, she fed her glandular system an abundance of fresh fruit and vegetable juices, as well as Seed Milk Supreme, until her glandular clocks were so youthfully adjusted, that the steady tick-tick-tick supply of rhythmic hormones made her look-feel . . . and *think young* again!

Seed Juices Regulate Hormone Health of Body. When seed juices or seed oils are used to nourish the body glands, they serve to regulate a rhythmic hormone flow to promote overall body-mind health. When the hormones are released in a steady balance, they serve to boost the ability of the heart, liver, kidney, brain, blood, and muscles. When they work to establish an internal "biological clock" through hormone harmony, they serve to nourish and boost the power of the brain through oxygen-hemoglobin enrichment. These same seed oils help in the assimilation and absorption of other fats that work to add a form of energy to the hormones, giving them the ability to continue their ceaseless internal washing and functioning.

To help improve glandular balance, seed oils as well as plant juices should play an important role in the quest for better health. It is said that the seed is a complete gland food; it contains within itself the factors of equilibrium and balance that are taken up by the hormones to create emotional and physical stability.

Plant and seed juices, in combination, offer a source of glandular food that may well be the all-natural source for the "think young" tonics which have always been sought. Nature offers these natural juices to help improve the pituitary-adrenals and related family of glands to issue forth the rhythmic stream of healthy and mentally rejuvenating hormones—"brain foods" from nature!

Summary

1. Fruit and vegetable juices are foods for the brain-boosting pituitary gland hormones.

2. Seed juices or seed oils help maintain internal cleanliness and promote oxygenation and better thinking processes.

3. Natural hormone tonics offer six special "think young" benefits.

4. Special "hormone tonics" helped Rose C. "think young" again.

5. A simple corrective program helps adjust the biological gland clocks.

6. A Brain Drink helped others enjoy better emotional health.

7. Seed milks helped Lillian I. enjoy hormone-nourished brain rejuvenation.

7

European Secrets for
a "Feel Young for Life"
Program Through
Special Hormone Foods

In Europe, the healthful practice of feeding the glands through natural nourishment has been followed for over a century. The great "back to nature" health spas and sanatoriums have long featured simple, quick, and surprisingly effective gland-feeding programs as a means of improving the health of the mind and body. These same programs have been prescribed for home use by the doctors of these European healing resorts, and many people have reported a feeling of rejuvenation when these unique programs alerted and revived their glandular networks. The special benefit of the European programs is attributed to just one word—*natural*. The European healers have always emphasized a *natural* approach as a means of helping the body's glands become properly adjusted to a rhythmic flow of youth-bestowing, healing hormones. These same all-natural programs may well be the ticket to a "feel young for life" benefit through hormone-energizing methods.

The Swiss Hormone Tonic That Helps Alert the Biological Gland Clocks to Boost Youthful Health

The famous Bircher-Benner Health Spa of Switzerland has long suggested the use of a unique but highly effective Swiss Hormone

Tonic as a means of helping to alert and adjust the biological gland clocks, so they can issue forth a steady, powerful supply of the hormones that boost youthful health. Many of the Bircher-Benner guests experienced hormone rejuvenation through this Tonic to such a high degree that they wanted to follow the same program at home, and it was suggested they make this quick-easy-effective gland food:

SWISS HORMONE TONIC. Obtain one pound of organic, shelled sunflower seeds, one-quarter pound of organic almonds, and one pound of organic wheat germ. Grind everything in a blender until a fine powder is left. *Next:* blend powder with a quart of milk and two tablespoons of organic honey.

Directions: Drink one glass of the Swiss Hormone Tonic in the morning, a second glass at noon (no other food is taken, since this Tonic reportedly has all the nourishing-satisfying nutrients of an average lunch), a third glass at dinnertime (your dinner should consist exclusively of a raw vegetable salad), and a final glass as a nightcap.

Benefits to Glandular Clocks: The *combination* of the high protein, vitamins, minerals, and enzymes work together to boost digestion and help feed the glands. The blending of these hormone food nutrients creates what is known as a "complete protein pattern" that is easily assimilated by the glandular system; these same nutrients in this unique "complete protein pattern" then become part of the hormones that go streaming directly into the circulatory system. In this complete pattern, the digested proteins or amino acids, are able to wind up and stimulate the sluggish gland clocks, so that a rhythmic balance of youth-building hormones helps improve the mind-body processes.

Swiss Hormone Tonic Becomes Wonder Healer. In one reported situation, Elsa R. came to the Bircher-Benner Spa, feeling rundown and prematurely aged (cold hands and feet, jagged nerve responses), displaying the symptoms of a completely rundown biological gland clock system.

Elsa R. reportedly had tried other programs, yet her health continued to decline. An understanding friend suggested that her endocrine glands were probably sluggish and that a return to nature would help alert them to a youthful hormone rhythm. Elsa R. was recommended to the Spa.

Raw Foods and Swiss Hormone Tonic—Simple, Effective. Her program consisted of lots of fresh air, rest, and controlled sunshine—

and her food program was that of exclusively raw hormone foods and the Swiss Hormone Tonic, every single day, as outlined above.

It was simple, yet effective. In three months' time, Elsa R. ate raw fruits, raw vegetables, and raw whole grains, and she drank non-processed milk—*no cooked foods*! This enabled her digestive system to receive the nutritional power to then absorb the foods from the Swiss Hormone Tonic, which was used to create a shower of rhythmic, healing hormones in her tired endocrine glands. It took three months of this hormone food program until Elsa R. developed color in her cheeks, soothing emotional tranquility, better nerve responses, a feeling of youthful health. Her hormone invigoration made her feel young, inside and outside. This invigoration is attributed to the "complete protein pattern" that is made available to the glandular clocks from hormone foods, to enable them to tick forth a healthful supply of youth-giving hormones. In combination with a raw and uncooked hormone food program, Elsa R. now felt the true joy of living! It is hoped that she still continues with the Swiss Hormone Tonic, even after it was suggested that she return to cooked meats, fish, and eggs, but with an emphasis on raw fruits and vegetables and whole grains.

Others who have had their glandular clocks adjusted by means of a raw hormone food program and the mandatory Swiss Hormone Tonic, daily, have experienced a marvelous return to youth! Many follow the programs at home—a simple set of programs which call for:

1. Daily, eat raw fruits, vegetables, grains.
2. Daily, drink the four glasses of the Swiss Hormone Tonic.
3. Daily, obtain sufficient rest, exercise, and healthful sleep.
4. For cooked foods, use fat-trimmed meats, high-protein salt-water fish (nothing frozen, nothing canned), fertile eggs, and non-processed dairy products. All foods should be as natural as possible, in the original state.

Simple? Yes. Effective? Overwhelmingly so, when the gland clocks are adjusted by all-natural means.

The Bavarian "Hormone Nourishment" Program

Father Sebastian Kneipp initiated a new century of natural

"hormone nourishment" by instructing his guests (he had a number of health spas and natural-healing sanatoriums throughout the province of Bavaria, as well as nearby states at the turn of the century) to follow a simple 15-step program. The benefit of this program is that it is soothingly healing to the glandular network; it offers a gradual adjustment so that the glands can then issue forth a healthful supply of youth-building hormones.

The 15-step program was so successful for thousands of followers of the natural healer, Father Kneipp, that it was taken up by other European spas and is still in use today. Many persons have built this program into their daily living and have found that it is simple, effective, and helps to keep the glands working in a healing manner. Here is the Father Kneipp "Hormone Nourishment Program," which requires *no* special apparatus, *no* complicated processes, *no* deprivation of any sort. It's easy, enjoyable, and hormone nourishing:

1. *Eat slowly.* Thoroughly chew your food to release the natural supply of nutrients that are needed by the glands as a form of nourishment so they can create a healthful supply of hormones. Hastily gulped food means that many of the nutrients cannot get to the glands, resulting in "starved" glands. Eat and chew comfortably and slowly.

2. *Be of good cheer.* While eating, do *not* permit any disturbing thoughts or actions to take place. Your glands function more healthfully when your emotional pattern is cheerful and optimistic. An angry thought or word creates a "tightening" reaction in the digestive system and an erratic gland clock mechanism. Be happy while eating—or else postpone a meal until you can feel cheerful.

3. *Eat foods that are gland satisfying.* If a certain food is disliked—mentally and/or physically—avoid it! Each person's glandular makeup is as personal and individual as his fingerprints. The most nutritious and healthful food for one person may be distasteful to another. To create gland harmony, eat foods that you find satisfying. If a healthful food is unappetizing to you for personal reasons, then substitute with another healthful food that *is* appetizing.

4. *Drink healthful beverages.* Your glands will be soothingly nourished with natural herb teas, fresh fruit and vegetable juices, and coffee substitutes. Eliminate the use of harsh coffee or tea which contain caffeine or tannic acids and other volatile oils. These whip up the action of the glands, causing internal frenzy and erratic hormone

function. Soda pop drinks are also taboo because of their caffeine and chemical content. Soothe your glands with honey-flavored natural herb teas, raw juices, and coffee substitutes.

5. *Drink water to please your thirsty glands.* Natural spring water offers a treasure of minerals needed to satisfy the "taste buds" of your thirsty glands. It also helps keep the glands lubricated. The same minerals and other nutrients contained in water help make up a river of healing and youth-building hormones. Father Kneipp recommended up to eight glasses of water daily. Natural spring water pleases the connective tissues of the glands, sparking them to issue forth enriched hormones that offer healing benefits to the body.

6. *Mornings, eat two whole apples and drink two glasses of water.* The glands function more efficiently when the digestive system is regularly cleansed of accumulated debris. In the morning, *on an empty stomach,* eat the two ripe apples (organic apples are suggested, but if unavailable, wash fresh apples under free-flowing, cold tap water to help dispose of possible pesticide-chemical sprays; some peeling may be done if you are concerned about insecticide residue), then drink the two glasses of room-temperature water. If from the tap, let the water stand a few moments so that it is comfortably cool. Bottled spring water that is natural is preferable, if available. *Benefit:* The minerals and enzymes in the fruit are taken up by the water, nourished by the glands, and then work to help create a natural bowel movement. This "internal scrubbing" of the vital organs and body's endocrine glands, helps them prepare for the day's hormone manufacturing processes.

7. *Liquids should be comfortably cool or comfortably hot.* All beverages should be gland-soothing. Ice-cold liquids are to be avoided because they constrict the delicate tubules and cellular networks of the glands, interfering with their effective hormone production ability. Excessively hot liquids may scorch and burn the sensitive linings of the internal tissues and harm the delicate gland tissues. Liquids should always be comfortably moderate in temperature.

8. *Fat-trimmed meat should be eaten thrice weekly.* Father Kneipp explained that meat has a high acid supply; also, meat contains uric acid which may impart a "burning" sensation to the glands. The substances and extractives in meat enter into the digested amino acids and find their way into the hormones to create a corrosive action on the body's organs. Father Kneipp felt that meat should be eaten no more than thrice weekly, that it should be fat trimmed, prepared by baking or broiling, and *never fried*! This

offered an amount of acid as well as animal protein that could be comfortably accommodated by the endocrine gland system.

9. *Eat fresh, ripe fruit and vegetables daily.* The raw food program was the basis for hormone stimulation in nearly all of the European health spas, notably those conducted by Father Kneipp. Raw fruits and vegetables—eaten separately—offer a tremendous source of vitamins, minerals, enzymes, and unsaturated fatty acids, as well as appreciable amounts of non-meat amino acids, which furnish "fuel" to the endocrine glands so they can then issue forth a healthful amount of hormones. *Raw* fruits and vegetables were the rule.

10. *Your bath water should be comfortably warm or cool—NEVER hot, NEVER ice cold.* Either extreme of boiling hot or freezing cold is regarded as shocking to the gland system. Father Kneipp had his patients take comfortably warm or cool tub or shower baths.

11. *Tobacco is to be eliminated.* The glands need breathing room! Tobacco tars and nicotine acids create a thick, heavy "cloud" in the system—*internal pollution*—that chokes off the vital breathing spaces for the glands. This reduces their efficiency. A return to the "feel young for life" program through natural hormones calls for the elimination of tobacco in any form.

12. *Alcoholic beverages are to be eliminated.* The scorching effects of alcohol can be deleterious to your glands. Alcohol is taken up by the pancreas and other glands, subjecting the delicate tissues to burning and depletion. The glands cast off the alcohol into the bloodstream, thereby creating further internal ill health. Father Kneipp and other natural healers insisted that alcohol be totally eliminated from the diet, as a means of helping the body nourish the glands to boost youthful hormones.

13. *Let your glands enjoy nightly rest.* The glands, along with other body organs and the five senses, require nightly rest. At least eight hours is reportedly soothing to the glands, easing their work load, enabling them to "nap," so they awaken refreshed and youthfully energetic the next morning. Sleep is "nourishment" for the glands.

14. *Relax your way to better gland function.* During the day, take small naps or "rest breaks" to help relax rising peaks of tension. In this manner, your biological clocks are able to go ticking ahead at a steady and hormonal rhythmic pace. If you're "all wound up," then hormone production is either excessive or sluggish because of nervous glands! You will find your health improving if you take occasional relaxation breaks and give your glands a little rest.

15. *A cheerful mind makes a cheerful hormone!* The adrenal and pituitary glands join with the thyroid and the rest of the endocrine family, to help boost your health—if you have a cheerful mind. *These glands are especially sensitive to emotional unrest.* A negative attitude, a mind that is filled with hatred, jealousy, anger, vengeance, and distrust, is one that causes the glands to react most shockingly. Often, a negative or hateful attitude can so wind up and distort the biological gland clocks that the hormone rhythm is seriously disrupted for days or weeks. The end result is impaired health. Father Kneipp was careful to note any gloom or depression amongst his guests, and he would gently suggest that they ally themselves with nature and be happy and cheerful—to help create equally happy glands and cheerful hormones.

Three Basic Benefits of the Bavarian "Hormone Nourishment" Program: Father Kneipp reported that this all-natural hormone food program brought about a marvelous healing through healthy hormones and offered these three basic benefits:

1. The Program helped the glands become *self-regulating.*
2. The Program enabled the glands to *self-adjust* to the rhythm of daily activities and to promote a youthful flow of healing hormones.
3. The Program enabled the precision-timed, adjusted gland clocks to bring about *self-rebuilding* through youthful hormones.

In review, the Program offered an opportunity for the glands to become self-regulating, self-adjusting, self-rebuilding! Youth through hormones was the successful reason behind Father Sebastian Kneipp's "Hormone Nourishment Program."

"ENTERS AN AGED PERSON...LEAVES AS A YOUNG PERSON." In one reported case study, Bertha J., at age 42, entered the Kneipp Spa, with reported feelings of complete physiological breakdown. She had a coated tongue, chronic cough, painful indigestion, chronic constipation, and a serious gall bladder disorder. Bertha J. entered stooped over, her arms and legs stiff, her eyes glazed, her complexion a waxen pallor. Father Kneipp thought she was double her 42 years of age.

Immediate Program Offered Partial Recovery. Under close supervision, Bertha J. was put on this special program. In particular, she was given a special Gland Broth that she was to take twice daily, at 2:00 p.m. and then at 6:00 p.m. Here is the recipe:

GLAND BROTH. In a stainless steel cooking utensil (no aluminum), place three cups grated raw carrots, three cups finely chopped celery, one cup chopped lettuce, and one-half cup chopped parsley or watercress.

Fill with one quart of natural spring water. Bring to a slow heat. *Do not boil.* When the Gland Broth steams, turn the heat very low. Simmer for 20 minutes. Stir frequently. Strain through cheese cloth or fine strainer. Squeeze out all the liquid. This is your Gland Broth.

Benefits: A treasure of minerals, especially potassium, offers "life's blood" to the malnourished glandular system. This mineral regulates the activity of the glands, helping them issue forth a rhythmic supply of youthful hormones. The potassium in this Gland Broth was the key to eventual correction of malfunctioning glands.

Recovery Noted in Three Weeks. When Bertha J. followed the closely supervised 15-step program and drank the Gland Broth twice daily, she experienced a remarkable recovery. Her limbs became youthfully flexible, her digestion improved, her five senses were more alert, her complexion cleared up, her skin had a healthful bloom. Bertha J. could actually see the years *roll back in time* when her gland clocks were properly adjusted. She was well on the way to recovery.

The Waerland Way of "Youth Through Hormones"

The Scandinavian healer, Are Waerland, brought a vital healing message to thousands who came to his health resorts in Sweden. Dr. Are Waerland offered a hormone-energizing program that reportedly was able to remedy so-called incurable problems and help promote a return to youth—through glandular rehabilitation!

Simple Secret: Dr. Are Waerland felt that the body's glands could be rehabilitated to gush forth youthful hormones *only when the errors of daily living were corrected*! His secret was to aim at curing the sick glands! Once this was accomplished through natural means, the healthy glands would then function smoothly to issue forth a rhythmic supply of life- and health-building hormones. "The life of the body is in the life of the glands," was his theme.

The Simple Gland Rehabilitation Program of Dr. Waerland

This Swedish healer reportedly healed tens of thousands of people by offering this *very simple* Gland Rehabilitation Program:

1. Foods should be natural and health-boosting and prepared in the home. No canned or processed foods of any kind were to be eaten.

2. Lots of fresh air, day and night, country walks, controlled sunshine exposure.

3. Exercise and physical activity every single day. Even ordinary walking or mild doctor-approved hiking was considered a healthful exercise.

4. Comfortable baths and vigorous body rubbing with a coarse towel helped stimulate sluggish nerve cells, which then helped boost gland-hormone responses.

5. Lots of raw fruits and vegetables and a lacto-vegetarian food program (he disapproved of meat and fish) as a means of providing nutrients to the glands, which are then used to make youthful hormones. NOTE: Dr. Waerland felt that meat and fish offer excessive uric acid that creates a corrosive hormone which is contrary to good health. Many of his followers experienced rejuvenation through a lacto-vegetarian program (fruits, vegetables, dairy products, eggs, seeds, nuts, etc.), and still many more reported rejuvenation on a once-a-week meat and/or fish program. Dr. Waerland preferred dietary elimination of meat and fish, but if this caused discomfort, then it was allowed in the interests of helping create emotional satisfaction.

6. A healthful mental attitude was needed to help create healthful glands. Dr. Waerland observed that the glands reacted either positively or negatively to emotional stimuli. He felt that nourishment could rehabilitate the glands—but emotions could cause upheaval. His followers were told to avoid arguments, competitive strain, and nervous unrest. This would help establish "glandular equilibrium" and promote a healthful environment.

Results: Thousands reported their biological gland clocks became so precision-timed that the youthful hormones helped heal their problems when other methods failed. In truth, Dr. Are Waerland was able to help the body heal itself—through glandular healing!

THE SWEDISH "FOREVER YOUTHFUL" HORMONE ELIXIR. In his healing sanatorium, Dr. Waerland created a special *morning elixir* that reportedly worked wonders in helping to nourish the glands and boost youthful hormones. Here is the simple recipe:

1 cup of vegetable juice
1 tablespoon whole flaxseed
1 teaspoon wheat bran

Let soak about 15 minutes. Stir well. Drink entirely—flaxseed and all. *Unique Benefit:* In the morning, the metabolic responses are slow and can react most favorably to this "Forever Youthful" Hormone Elixir. The vegetable juice is rich in minerals that are taken up by the unsaturated fatty acids of the seeds and given power-plus in the task of awakening and rehabilitating the glands.

The "Forever Youthful" Hormone Elixir is *alkaline* in reaction, neutralizing excess acidosis, helping to dispel those "bubbles" that cause internal bloating. The flaxseed is a healing herb that has long been used by herbalists as a means of soothing glandular unrest.

In combination with the other nutrients, this "Forever Youthful" Hormone Elixir may well be the European "secret" for glandular rehabilitation.

WAERLAND "HAPPY HORMONE" PROGRAM. In brief, the way to rehabilitate the glands and issue forth "happy hormones" is to ally yourself with nature. Dr. Waerland told his followers they were to *eliminate* sharp spices or condiments, including salt, vinegar, pepper, ketchup, and mustard. No coffee, tea, alcohol, or tobacco were allowed. No white sugar or white flour, or any products made with these bleached items, could be used. No canned, refined, chemically processed, or treated foods were allowed. OPTIONAL: No eating of meat or fish allowed. Dr. Waerland noted his followers had better glandular rehabilitation on a meatless and fishless food program. Many others who ate meat and fish—once a week for each—also experienced glandular improvement, which suggests that this could be optional.

For tens of thousands in the past and currently in Europe, the popular Waerland System has helped rehabilitate the glands and boost the rhythm of youthful hormones—the natural way.

Many of the reported European programs are finding their way into American lives, helping the body's processes become rehabilitated and giving the body and mind an opportunity to enjoy a renewed youth—through "forever young" glands and hormones. The "back to nature" movement is effective in helping one's health become boosted and improved—through nature.

Unique Chapter Highlights

1. The Bircher-Benner Health Spa program can easily be followed in your own home. Begin with the Swiss Hormone Tonic.

2. The 15-step program outlined by Father Sebastian Kneipp, the miracle healer from Bavaria, helps remake and readjust the gland clocks, promoting healthful hormones.

3. The Gland Broth offers a powerhouse of nourishment to the glands.

4. The Scandinavian gland rehabilitation program, created by Dr. Are Waerland, brought renewed youth to tens of thousands of people.

5. The Swedish "Forever Youthful" Hormone Elixir, when taken in combination with the six basic steps outlined by Dr. Waerland, helps glands issue forth "happy hormones" and life that is brimming with youth.

8

How to Enrich Your Bloodstream for Youthfulness with Hormone Foods

A youthful bloodstream needs to be "washed" until it is sparkling clean. The cleansing action is performed by an inter-related movement of all of the body glands. When properly adjusted with an iron-rich food program, the glands are able to issue forth a supply of nourishing hormones which pour directly into the bloodstream, performing a rhythmic washing-enrichment that helps promote a look and feel of energetic youthfulness. Because the bloodstream receives its nourishment *directly* from the hormones, it is essential to provide your glands with a healthful and natural supply of nutrients, which help bring about this rhythmic washing-enrichment process that goes on throughout the entire lifespan. If the glands are maladjusted, if the hormones are "thin" or deprived of adequate vitality, then the bloodstream becomes less effective in helping to boost body and mind health. In brief, healthy hormones bring nutrition directly to the bloodstream. Hormones are often regarded as the "fountains" which empty directly into the bloodstream to help wash and enrich the rivers of life. A properly nourished "fountain" will gush forth a treasure of health into these running rivers. The hormone fountains are as nourished as the glands, themselves. It is all part of the inter-related rhythmic movement that occurs in your body. The source of power is basically that of proper nourishment and assimilation of nutrients from foods.

The Mineral That Adjusts the Blood-Building Glands

One food mineral has been seen to have the natural power of being able to adjust the thyroid-adrenal-parathyroid glands so that they are able to issue a fresh and energetic supply of hormones that will help boost the quality of the bloodstream and also help improve basic body health. That food mineral is *iron.*

How Iron Invigorates Healthy Hormones for the Bloodstream. When iron is metabolized, the glands use it to manufacture the vital red blood cells in the bone marrow. The glands then take the iron and put it in their hormones, which are later used to help the cells carry oxygen from the lungs to the other body parts; the hormones energize the red blood cells to transport waste products back to the lungs to be exhaled. This is part of the self-cleansing action that "washes" the bloodstream and also helps promote basic blood health. Glandular hormones are likened unto nature's own "internal nuclear energy," in that they promote this rhythmic movement of the bloodstream to help maintain and improve body health.

Hormones deposit valuable iron into the bloodstream; once this mineral is present, the blood flows into the body tissues and transports excessive wastes and sludge, which must be removed, thereby helping to create the life-giving processes of daily living.

Iron offers energy to the glandular network to propel the blood and causes it to act in much the same manner as an internal conveyor system. Namely, the hormone-powered bloodstream extracts the "raw materials" provided by the glands and goes streaming throughout the entire network of arteries, capillaries, and veins, helping to put roses into your cheeks, build resistance against infection, promote better healing, nourish the other glands and vital body organs, boost energy, and clear up thinking processes. This entire process is sparked when the food mineral, *iron,* is made available by the assimilative processes of the glands. An iron-poor hormone means an iron-poor bloodstream! To help provide your bloodstream with much-needed iron, begin with feeding your glands.

How James T. Boosted Iron-Rich Blood Cells with Natural Foods

Fatigue made James T. walk and sit with stooped shoulders, wear a sweater in warm weather, feel cold, and have clammy hands and feet. His sallow complexion was a clue to the iron deficiency in his hormone rivers. James T. caught one cold after another, developed allergic symptoms, and felt rundown and chronically tired even if he would have a night's sleep. While he felt his natural food program was adequate, he was told to boost his supply of iron, which was needed by the adrenal-thyroid glands as well as the others, in order to help provide a rich supply of mineral-nourished hormones that empty directly into the bloodstream. Here is the simple, effective, all-natural, iron-feeding hormone tonic that he took, each morning:

IRON-FEEDING HORMONE TONIC: Buy sun-dried and *unsulphured* apricots (usually found at health stores). Put a handful of this natural fruit in the bottom of a deep dish. Cover with some slightly boiled water. Stir. Cover the dish. Let remain until cool. Then place in the refrigerator overnight. *In the morning:* pour the apricot juice into a glass and drink slowly. You may also eat the fruit as part of your breakfast. NOTE: You may also use sun-dried and *unsulphured* peaches, raisins, or prunes, singly or in combination.

BENEFITS: James T. found that this Iron-Feeding Hormone Tonic helped improve his blood health by offering these benefits:

1. The glands needed the iron to send to the bone marrow, where they helped transform it into a form that went into the red blood cells. The hormones then took the iron-rich blood cells out of the bone marrow to be sent gushing into the bloodstream, performing a much-needed washing and enrichment of the entire red network!

2. The iron in this all-natural tonic was used by the hormones to nourish the hemoglobin (red coloring matter of blood). In particular, the hormones used the iron to build and rebuild the four globin molecules found in each molecule of hemoglobin. The iron was needed to perform this internal self-renewal mechanism. The hormones functioned as efficiently as they could, depending upon the iron supply available.

3. The iron in this tonic worked with the hormones to take amino acids from the digestive system, which were used to strengthen the blood cell molecules. Each globin molecule contains all the essential amino acids and many non-essential amino acids. An iron-rich hormone is able to extract amino acids from the digestive system as building blocks for the molecules. But an iron-poor hormone is deficient and may not be able to process all of the amino acids to the bloodstream, and the globin molecules may thus become protein-starved. This is one link in the chain reaction of blood health decline

that leads to conditions of ill health. The key to blood enrichment is in the iron that boosts the glandular-hormone "magnetic action" to take up amino acids to use as foundation structures for the globin molecules.

4. The hormone-invigorated rivers in James T.'s bloodstream were like master builders of hemoglobin. The hormones used the iron to help create warmth, vitality, and natural stamina. The iron in the hormone tonic combined with other nutrients that helped create a full quota of top-quality red blood cells.

James T. Becomes "Young and Healthy" with Iron-Feeding Hormone Tonic. Each morning, James T. took this natural hormone food tonic. It helped improve his gland health so that the iron-carrying hormones could then promote better blood circulation and basic invigoration. His shoulders felt straight, his vision cleared, he had a tingling warmth in his fingers and toes, his complexion had a healthy sparkle, his allergies were less noticeable, and he felt "young and healthy" all over—thanks to the iron-fed hormones from the hormone food he consumed.

Your One-Day Gland-Feeding Program to Help Improve Blood Health

Here is a reported one-day corrective hormone food program that is tastefully delicious, uses natural foods, and offers a balanced supply of nutrients, as well as iron, which helps boost the biological gland clock activity and sends a stream of mineral-rich hormones directly into the iron-requiring bloodstream.

BEFORE BREAKFAST

Drink 2 glasses of Iron-Feeding Hormone Tonic.

BREAKFAST

2 eggs, poached or as you like them—soft- or hard-boiled
1 slice 100% whole-wheat bread
1 pat butter
2 tablespoons sun-dried, organically grown raisins
1 cup whole grain oatmeal
1 tablespoon wheat germ sprinkled on oatmeal
1 8-ounce glass of milk
1 medium orange, peeled

LUNCHEON

Small baked potato (eat jacket)
1/2 cup cooked greens
1 thin slice 100% whole-wheat bread
1 pat butter
Tossed vegetable salad—large bowl
1 8-ounce glass milk
2 tablespoons sun-dried, organically grown raisins

MID-AFTERNOON

1 8-ounce glass unsweetened grape juice

SUPPER

*1 serving (4 halves) apricots or peaches (2 halves) canned with water, no syrup.
1 thin slice 100% whole-wheat bread
1 pat butter
1 8-ounce glass of milk
1/2 cup cottage cheese
Vegetable soup or broth

*Note: Alternate fruits for supper, or have a mixed fruit salad for variety.

NIGHT CAP

Blackstrap molasses—1 tablespoon—in hot milk.

IRON SUPPLY: The preceding reported One-Day Gland-Feeding Program offers close to 30 milligrams of iron, that are speedily utilized by the glands and are then taken up by the hormones to be washed directly into the bloodstream. Just one day of careful dieting is involved, but it can make a world of difference for your health!

THE EVERYDAY FOOD THAT CONTROLS HORMONE IRON SUPPLY. A simple and tasty everyday food holds the key to the metabolization of iron. This food is used by the adrenals and thyroid, in rhythm with the pancreas, *to create an acid medium in which the iron is dissolved.* Because the glands can absorb iron *only* in an acid environment, they need this natural food as a means of performing the task of using iron for their hormones. To help create a healthful and natural acid media for the iron-metabolizing glands, you should partake of these foods daily:

Buttermilk, sour milk, yogurt, all citrus fruits, apples, and *tart* fruits.

Make Your Own Acid Medium. Ordinary sour milk, known

throughout Bulgaria and Europe for hundreds of years, is coming into its own recognition here in the United States as a food needed by the glands for its all-natural acid qualities. You can make your own acid medium by preparing homemade sour milk in this easy way:

Sour Milk: Place two tablespoons of lemon juice in one glass of milk and stir. Cover and let stand at room temperature until it becomes firm and custard-like. Refrigerate until ready to eat with a spoon.

Benefits: The Homemade Sour Milk offers a natural acid medium in the digestive system. This enables the hormones to dissolve iron from ingested foods, then use this mineral to help promote better blood and body health. It is healthful to drink one glass of Homemade Sour Milk every single day as a means of giving the glands the acid medium they require for iron metabolization.

THE SIMPLE PROGRAM THAT REJUVENATED A DE-SIGNER'S BLOODSTREAM. Janice E. worked as a dress designer and had to remain indoors for long periods of time. She looked pale and felt wan and listless. Her hands frequently trembled, and her once-strong fingers could not hold a needle as steadily as in her youth. (She was all of 39. She felt much older.) Janice E. had recurring problems of indigestion. She was also troubled with constipation and occasional bouts of colitis. This caused a draining out of valuable nutrients as well as iron and was largely responsible for her "poor blood."

Uses Nature to Boost Gland Health. Janice E. used all-naturaι means to help revive her sluggish glandular condition. She would drink two glasses of Homemade Sour Milk every single day. She boosted her citrus fruit intake and also increased her iron supply. In particular, she found this simple recipe helped her glandular network become iron-sparked with blood-washing powers:

Liver 'n' Wheat Germ. She would dip liver in wheat germ, coating the liver. Then she would broil the liver in vegetable oil. This provided her with a supply of iron, protein, and the valuable B-complex vitamins. Now Janice's glands had "fuel" from which to help in the iron metabolism.

Rejuvenation Hits Stumbling Block. Janice's gland-feeding program helped boost her blood health, made her feel warm and alert, improved her complexion, and put color back into her lips and fingernails. Once her iron-rich hormones washed and bathed her bloodstream, she was less susceptible to colds and sniffles and lesser allergies. But—her rejuvenation hit a stumbling block. She had recurring and repeating bouts with chronic diarrhea as well as constipation (symptoms of colitis). This drained out the precious iron sources and her glands were denied sufficient amounts of this mineral. She began to slide back.

Antacids-Laxatives Cause Glandular Unrest. Janice E. took frequent antacids to ease digestive burning sensations. She further abused her hormones by taking laxatives to ease occasional constipation. A problem arose because the antacids depleted the needed acid medium for iron metabolization; the laxatives whipped up the intestinal network to expel wastes as well as to expel needed nutrients. As a consequence, the hormones were denied much of their valuable B-complex, iron, and protein nourishment. Small wonder she started to slide back.

All-Natural Hormone Food Program Adjusts Biological Gland Clocks. Janice E. felt encouraged by her partial blood rejuvenation, so she returned to an all-natural program to help correct the maladjusted biological gland clocks. She eliminated artificial foods, salt, pepper, spices, sugar, and white flour, as well as foods made from them. This helped soothe the fluttering glandular reactions. Gradually, as her endocrine glands were properly adjusted, her natural acid supply was sufficient to enable the hormones to perform their dissolving action upon ingested iron. Now the metabolized iron could be used by the hormones to help wash the bloodstream, pep up and boost its power, and promote healthful living. Janice E. felt healthfully young again—thanks to adjusted gland clocks and iron-rich hormones in her bloodstream!

How to Feed Iron to Your Glands

Wholesome, natural, and healthful foods that have good iron supplies are these: desiccated liver, turnips, greens, soybeans, blackstrap molasses, liver, meat, mushrooms, sunflower seeds, eggs, heart, kidney, and lentils. NOTE: One average slice of calves' liver offers as much as 21 milligrams of iron! One cup of non-processed wheat bran will offer as much as 12 milligrams of iron!

Dark-Colored Juices Boost Iron Supply in Hormones. Dark-colored grape juice, or the juice of any dark fruit, such as blackberries, blueberries, currants, raisins, or plums, help the glands increase the iron supply available to the hormones that further boost the production of red blood cells.

Suggestion: Drink one glass of dark-colored berry juice twice daily. *Benefits:* The iron is taken up by the glands, metabolized, and put into the hormones. These hormones then wash the bloodstream and enrich the rivers of life with the hemoglobin-making iron to promote the making and storage of iron in the bone marrow. The iron-carrying hormones in the bloodstream then have a favorable benefit upon the tiny capillaries throughout the entire body. To maintain this rhythmic hormone balance, iron must be present in the system. Feed your glands a daily amount of healthful iron from berry juices.

THE SIMPLE FOOD THAT STRENGTHENS THE HORMONES TO PROTECT THE BLOOD CELLS. Lecithin, one of the phospholipids (fat-melting) food products made from soybeans, is an essential nutrient for the hormones. The well-nourished hormones use lecithin to create an "envelope" wrapped around the blood corpuscles, preventing them from undue destruction. The hormones need lecithin, which is then used to make this protective envelope for the blood cells. *Where to Obtain Lecithin:* It is available as a powder or in granules at most health food stores. Sprinkle in a glass of vegetable juice and have a healthful, hormone-strengthening food. Since the original source of lecithin is the soybean, it is gland food that should be part of your regular eating program to build better blood health. Serve soybeans regularly as a main or side dish, accompanying healthful foods.

Blood-Building, "Forever Young" Gland Brew

In a cup of freshly prepared, dark green vegetable juice, stir four tablespoons of desiccated liver (the dehydrated form of liver, with fat and connective tissues removed, sold at most health food stores), two tablespoons of powdered lecithin, and two tablespoons of Brewer's Yeast powder. Sprinkle with sea salt for a tangy flavor. Stir vigorously. (For best results, try to buzz in a blender for just one minute.) Drink this Blood-Building, "Forever Young" Gland Brew and derive these health-helping benefits:

1. The high iron content is taken up by the endocrine glands, sparked by the B-complex vitamins in the yeast and energized by the minerals in the vegetable juice. This combination of factors enables the glands to help metabolize nutrients to make them more readily assimilated by the bloodstream.

2. The Brew will help deposit a healthful supply of oxygen in the hemoglobin, enabling the hormone-enriched rivers of life to flow from head to toe, boosting basic health.

3. A unique action of the Vitamin B12 in the desiccated liver helps to boost an *intrinsic* factor—this is something that the glands create *inside* the digestive system, which cannot come from anything *extrinsic* or outside. Namely, the endocrine glands use the Vitamin B12 to work in with the iron and minerals to enrich the hormones so they can then carry the metabolized nutrients right into the bloodstream. In turn, the healthful, hormone-enriched bloodstream is now able to bring about the rejuvenation of the cells and tissues, organs, and muscle cells. This *intrinsic* factor is sparked by the inter-relationship of the nutrients in the all-natural, hormone food Blood-Building, "Forever Young" Gland Brew, working to send a healthful supply of blood to all cells, tissues, the liver, bone marrow, spleen, and other glands and organs.

4. The Brew helps iron combine with the hemoglobin; then the hormones prompt the iron to float freely through the bloodstream, promoting a cleansing action, filling the entire lifestream with youthful invigoration. The enriched hormones see to it that one-half of the body's iron supply is in motion in the bloodstream; the other half is stored in the body's organs. NOTE: This rhythmic pattern is made possible when the endocrine glands are properly "computerized" with the all-natural programs described herein.

In Brief: The Blood-Building, "Forever Young" Gland Brew offers a rich supply of those necessary elements that become "fuel" for the endocrines to enable them to issue forth a blood-washing supply of healthful lifestreams.

The hormones have the power to create good vs. poor absorption of nutrients into the bloodstream. Give your hormones their much-needed power with healthful hormone food programs.

Because the life of a red blood cell is from 40-120 days, it is necessary to have a healthful and vigorously working, iron-rich hormone supply available to make up for the losses. As fast as these red blood cells disintegrate, there must be a supply of iron-rich hormones standing by to help manufacture a set of new cells. This is part of the rhythmic clock-ticking hormone supply that is made possible through good, healthful practices.

BANANAS BOOST HORMONE ABSORPTION ABILITIES. It is reported that bananas are helpful to the glands in boosting their absorption abilities. The iron in the banana energizes the glands to issue those hormones which cause regeneration of hemoglobin. All of the iron in the banana is used by the hormones for forming hemoglobin. This tree-ripened fruit is unique in that the hormones readily utilize its available form of iron as well as other minerals and nutrients.

Suggestion: In a bowl of whole grain cereal, add several slices of banana and a dark fruit and sprinkle with wheat germ and sun-dried raisins. Give your hormones a powerhouse of "metabolic force" to enable them to use the iron to help make, remake, regenerate, and rehabilitate the bloodstream, promoting a feeling of vital energy.

A Hormone-Washed Bloodstream Is the Key to Youthful Health. The endocrine glands need to be alerted, adjusted, and precision timed by means of healing foods, to enable them to issue forth a supply of hormones that work to wash the bloodstream, promote a youthful mind and body, and help instill a love of life and health!

Important Chapter Highlights

1. The bloodstream receives nourishment *directly* from the hormones. To help wash and rejuvenate your bloodstream, your hormones should be healthfully nourished.

2. Iron is the "star mineral" that adjusts the biological blood-building glands to issue forth stimulating hormones.

3. An all-natural program boosted iron-rich blood cells for James T.

4. Start the day right by alerting your sleepy glands with an Iron-Feeding Hormone Tonic.

5. Just a One-Day Gland-Feeding Program helps start your glands on the way to healthful blood-feeding hormones.

6. Iron dissolves in an acid medium. Try the listed homemade sour milk and other foods to help your hormones create a healthful acid medium for iron metabolization.

7. Janice E. followed a simple rejuvenation program that boosted her blood health. Liver 'n' Wheat Germ, Homemade Sour Milk, and natural foods helped improve her glandular rhythm.

8. One simple food, lecithin, causes a built-in, self-protective mechanism used by hormones to shield red blood cells from premature aging.

9. The Blood-Building, "Forever Young" Gland Brew creates hormone harmony when used in conjunction with basic natural health programs.

10. Tasty bananas may offer energy to the glands to issue forth healthful hormones.

9

How Food Hormones in Fruits Help Free You from Aging Allergies

Nature has placed a treasure trove of allergy-resisting food hormone substances in fresh, raw fruits, to help the body build resistance to allergies. These substances are like "fruit hormones," in that they are the life's blood of the fruit, bringing about its own plant metabolism and good health, as well as freedom from infection, when grown in harmony with natural principles. In particular, *tree-ripened stone fruits* are a prime source of the hormones that are used by the body's endocrine gland system as a supplement to its own hormones. The hormones in these stone fruits are prime sources of the ingredients that then go to make up the body's own hormones, helping build resistance to allergies and also promoting relief from allergic upset.

How Stone Fruit Hormones Ease Allergic Distress. Stone-bearing fruits develop from naturally pollinated flowers. They are tree ripened and are usually in season until they are ripe. During this natural ripening process, the pollination causes a complete fruit metabolization. The natural process changes the starches into a form of sugar that is rich in levulose and in a state of complete digestion, that is taken up speedily by the body's glands to send to the bloodstream in the form of hormones, to help build resistance to infections and allergic symptoms.

Stone fruits are naturally sweet and pre-digested by their own hormones during the ripening process, making it easy for your own gland system to accept the healthful ingredients.

Stone fruit hormones (in the form of levulose and natural fruit sugar hormones) have been pre-digested, thereby sparing your own endocrine system the energy-expending effort of metabolization. This offers your hormones a healthful and "speedy" supply of fruit hormones, saving your glands tiresome effort and enabling your hormones to be fed by the fruit's own hormones.

Stone Fruits Which Have "Speedy" Food Hormones: Look for any seasonal fruit that has a large stone or pit. This is your guide to nature-pollinated fruits with pre-digested hormones. Good selections include: dates, mangos, papayas, apricots, peaches, avocados, cherries, plums, prunes, and grapes (with seeds, regarded as stones or pits and evidence of natural ripening). Always select *seasonal* fruits and those which are *naturally ripe.* This is your guide to the nature-created digestion of the fruit and its available supply of its own hormones. This pre-digested levulose hormone will then help boost the power of your body's hormones.

How Hormone Foods Controlled and Healed Allergies

Ralph J. was a longtime victim of hay fever and allergies, and he suffered bouts with asthma as well. While medication offered periodic relief from symptoms, there were year-round recurring attacks of hay fever and food allergies, as well as asthma. In the latter case, the asthma had been so severe, that there was the threat of bronchitis as well as permanent respiratory injury. Ralph J. then went on a special "fruit hormone" program. It was surprisingly simple and all-natural, but reportedly so effective, that it was able to relieve Ralph's hay fever, allergies, and asthma.

Simple Fruit Hormone Program: Ralph J. would take daily amounts of fresh, seasonal, raw stone fruits! Each day, he would eat a fresh stone fruit salad with each of his meals. He would eat as much as was comfortably possible and deliciously enjoyable. The results? He reported that he experienced welcome relief from his allergic symptoms and appeared to be well on the way to a more permanent healing. The fruit hormones had created a natural antibiotic in Ralph's bloodstream, building resistance and cleansing benefits to ease sensitivity to allergic offenders. NOTE: Stone fruit hormones are said to have the capacity to aid in oxidation and fight infectious germs. Fruit hormones unite with body hormones to create a germ-fighting action that eases allergic sensitivities.

Ralph J. continued on with his fruit program until his own hormone system had become nourished sufficiently to be able to resist allergic distress. Hormone foods had helped him enjoy freedom from allergies.

Five Allergy-Easing Benefits of Stone Fruit Hormone Foods

During the pollination and tree-ripening pre-digestion process of stone fruits, the natural hormones in the fruits and their juices become metabolized so they contain substances which offer these five allergy-easing benefits:

1. *Fruit Hormones Nourish Body Glands and Tissues.* Stone fruit hormones are speedily soluble in the system and are oxidized to dehydro-ascorbic acid, which is then sent in high concentration to metabolically active body tissues: the retina, pituitary gland, adrenal cortex, thymus, liver, brain, testes, and ovaries. With this overall body enrichment of hormone foods, resistance to allergies is increased.

2. *Fruit Hormones Help Body Boost Its Own Resistance.* The natural fruit hormones coming into the body's own glandular system work to take part in many metabolic activities as co-factors. They serve both in reduction and oxidation of harmful infectious substances. The stone fruit hormones protect many vital enzymes and co-enzymes, along with other nutrients, against oxidation. This builds up the body's own reserves to resist allergic infections.

3. *Fruit Hormones Help Glands in Protein Metabolism.* The "secret" of fruit hormone power in helping resist allergies is in its ability to help the body glands in protein metabolism. Fruit hormones help to bring about assimilation of amino acids. One reaction of particular benefit is the hydro-oxylation of the amino acid, proline, into hydroxyproline. This particular amino acid is then sent by fruit hormones into the collagen fibers of connective tissues. The collagen is distributed throughout the intercellular spaces of the body, strengthening the tissues to resist breakdown, the first symptom of an allergic disorder. Fruit hormones assist in bringing about this manufacture of collagen (cement or glue to hold together tissues and cells) in order to resist colds, asthmatic symptoms, bronchial disorders, and hay fever.

4. *Fruit Hormones Regulate Body Hormones.* Stone fruit hor-

mones influence the body's glands and help regulate a rhythmic flow of allergy-resisting hormones. These same fruit hormones become involved in the adrenal gland release of cortisone to ease infectious sensitivities. The same fruit hormones stimulate the other glands to enhance the absorption of iron, to convert substances into a glandular secretion known as norepinephrine—a vital allergy-fighting neurohormone. It is, in effect, the same as using fruit hormones for nature's own medicines! The fruit hormones nourish the body glands to help pep up their function in fighting allergic symptoms.

5. *Fruit Hormones Boost Unique Body Hormone Action.* The pre-digested fruit hormones become involved in hydroxylation of tryptophan to form a substance which then helps the body's glands issue forth a neurohormone, serotonin. These powerful amino acids build the health of most body organs through the central and autonomic nervous systems. They cause a healthful body hormone rhythm that eases susceptibility to allergies. With the building and maintenance of collagenous supportive tissues, the steady flow of hormones are natural self-defenses against the ravages of infectious colds, allergies, and related disorders.

Stone Fruit Hormone Foods Promote Health Through Glandular Nourishment. A healthfully activated gland network will issue forth hormones that help grow or mend bones, heal blood vessels, promote internal knitting of broken cells and tissues, soothe the allergy-infected cartilage, improve energy, boost a healthful appetite, and offer "buffer hormones" against bacterial toxins of infection.

Once stone fruit have deposited their "buffer hormones" into the bloodstream, there is added protection against allergic infections; the "buffer hormones" promote healing, preserve enzyme activity, favor cellular proliferation, and aid tissue rejuvenation. *Most important: the stone fruit "buffer hormones" increase the body's resistance to common stresses, such as those caused by bacterial toxins, low temperature, and fatigue. By bringing about self-adjustment and self-regulation of healing hormones, stone fruits build resistance to allergic discomforts.*

FRUIT HORMONE FOODS HEAL PROBLEMS OF CHILLS, FEVER, AND HEAD COLD. In one reported case, Barbara J. had severe chills, fever, and a nagging head cold for upwards of 14 days. Nothing seemed to bring relief. She then developed a severe pounding headache that made her look and feel worse. Barbara J. was in despair until she was placed on a special, all-natural program that called for stimulating her glands to produce healing hormones.

The program called for large amounts of stone fruits. She would eliminate other foods that were high in sugar and made of white flour. This called for a soothing of the endocrine glands and eased their energy expenditure. Now the glands could be nourished by stone fruit hormones. The glands were invigorated by this all-natural "hormone supplement." Barbara J. was soon able to recover from the chills and fever. Her head cold symptoms eased. Her headache was gone.

The fruit hormones helped in the glandular process of oxidation, which made it a valuable germ-fighting reaction. The fruit hormones were regarded as all-natural "antibiotics" in being able to unite with the virus and help oxidate it through the skin pores, thus casting out the infectious allergy-causing offender. Fruit hormones helped bring about this action and promoted a healing for Barbara J.

Natural Hormone Food Program Promoted
Resistance to Dust Allergies

George T. was employed in a machine shop that was frequently infiltrated with offensive dust. George T. would sneeze, have running eyes and nose, and would sputter and choke. At times, his dust sensitivity was so great, that he would wheeze and choke, gasp for air, turn pale, and have to go outside to "catch a breath of air." This outside air was polluted and this further increased the sensitivity of his bronchial tubes. His situation grew worse as the factory dust increased in amount. For a while, George T. thought he might have to look for another job, since there was no way in which the machine shop could seal off the dust coming from the adjoining factory complex. George T. felt miserable and unhappy.

Builds Self-Resistance Through Natural Programs. When his allergies increased to food allergies, it turned out to be a blessing in disguise. He could not eat canned or processed foods because the additives irritated his already sensitive system. So he turned to natural and whole foods—particularly whole stone fruits. It was the start of a return to natural foods. In particular, George T. ate lots of fresh and seasonal, tree-ripened stone fruits. These included apricots, peaches, cherries, plums, and whatever else was available in a natural, tree-ripened supply. Soon, he found himself being able to resist many of his bronchial allergies.

How Hormone Foods Eased George's Bronchitis. The glands readily welcomed the supply of "buffer hormones" in the stone fruits to supplement their own rhythmic rivers. In particular, this is how fruit hormones eased bronchial allergic disorders for George:

The stone fruit hormones stimulated the adrenal glands to issue forth an extra supply of adrenalin, which was sent streaming into the bloodstream to help neutralize those toxins and bacterial infections which made George T. sensitive to dust offenders.

An *underactivity* of the adrenal glands means a deficiency of those hormones which serve the purpose of neutralizing wastes and nullifying the irritating effects of harsh bacterial infections. To correct this hormone slowdown, the stone fruit hormones were used as all-natural supplementation. Furthermore, nutrients in stone fruits served to invigorate and nourish the adrenals until they could issue forth a *healthful activity* of allergy-fighting hormones.

Unique Benefit: Because tree-ripened stone fruit hormones are available in a pre-digested levulose form, they are *immediately absorbed* into the bloodstream and go *speedily* to work to help promote bacterial cleansing and toxin fighting that will ease allergic symptoms.

FRUIT HORMONES SET UP BIOLOGICAL GLAND CLOCKS IN HORMONE RHYTHM. Fruit hormones assist the body's endocrine glands to set up a "clock rhythm" to help send forth a steady supply of allergy-resisting buffer zones. Fruit hormones join with body enzymes (natural proteins that carry out metabolic processes by which living things are digested into usable nutrients) to help the biological gland clocks become properly adjusted so they can send forth a rhythmic supply of healing hormones.

A unique benefit is that the fruit hormones help the body glands produce *controlled* hormone reactions, sending forth what is often regarded as a time-release process. Gradually, throughout the day and night, as you work, rest, and sleep, the fruit hormones offer a "time release" of allergy-fighting substances into the bloodstream. This offers a steady and rhythmic supply of these valuable allergy-easing hormones. *Benefit:* With a steady tick-tick-tick supply of such hormones, there is less problem of "middle of the night" bronchial attacks, less distressful "coughing-sneezing spells," and *more staying power through stone fruit hormone energizing.* Also, there is less "midday letdown" and less "night-time misery." During certain hours of the day or night, metabolism irregularities may also be the spark which ignites an allergic attack. But a natural way to help ease such problems is to follow the natural laws of healthful living and take advantage of the benefits of the *controlled hormone rhythm* established through stone fruits.

How to Help Fruit Hormones Nourish the Body Glands

The hormones in fresh stone fruit will have a more healthful vigor if they are favored with a natural internal environment. This calls for the following of a few very simple but highly effective hormone-boosting health plans:

1. *Emphasize wholesome, natural foods.* Your allergy-correcting food program should consist of wholesome, natural fruits, vegetables, meats, seeds, nuts, fish, and poultry. Eliminate packaged and artificially processed foods. These contain harsh chemicals and additives which interfere with glandular absorption of fruit hormones.

2. *Daily, eat a bowl of seasonal, fresh, raw stone fruit.* Build immunity through the daily eating of stone fruit. Do this at breakfast to help give the adrenals a good start in the morning. You might also have a "fruit break" in which you will eat luscious, succulent, tree-ripened stone fruit as a meal in itself. You could also finish meals with fruit for a metabolic digestive aid to hormone assimilation.

3. *Select a variety of other fruits to maintain balance.* Daily, eat other seasonal fresh, raw fruit in order to maintain dietary variety and balance. Other fruit is rich in natural vitamins, minerals, amino acids, enzymes, and some unsaturated fatty acids, which are needed by the glandular system to manufacture allergy-fighting hormones.

4. *Eliminate suspect allergic offenders.* Give your hormones a helping hand in fighting allergies by eliminating allergic offenders. Dispose of foods, fumes, chemicals, mold spores, and house dust which may be suspect as causing allergic unrest.

5. *Maintain healthful stimulation of glands through corrective nutrition.* Help adjust your gland clocks to healthful hormone stimulation by means of a boosted protein intake, increased minerals, as well as vitamins. These serve as "batteries" to boost the vigor of the glands to function in their hormone-issuing, allergy-fighting function.

6. *Fresh stone fruit juices offer hormone cleansing benefit.* The fresh juices of raw stone fruits are especially rich in nutrients and hormones which help correct the toxic effects of allergens; these "juice hormones" also help detoxify the harmful effects of allergens which have entered the blood, whether they be dusts, dandruff, foods, etc. Once these "juice hormones" have been poured into the bloodstream, they work to cleanse the system of infectious bacteria

and help ease problems such as stuffy nose, hay fever, asthma, eczema, hives, and related allergic symptoms. Hormones do make a difference!

7. *Stone fruit hormone foods help protect against outside infections.* These hormones work to build a mucilaginous substance which serves much in the same manner as cement does in a brick building, except that this "concrete" is in the form of a stiff jelly. The fruit hormones help build this stiff jelly or strong connective tissue to protect the body's cells and tissues and protect against the invasion of outside offenders and infectious bacteria. *Suggestion:* Help build up immunity to allergies by providing a daily supply of fresh, raw stone fruits with each meal. If you are susceptible to winter colds, bronchial disorders, asthmatic attacks, recurring sniffles, head colds, and related allergic problems, reach for raw stone fruits, and help feed your glands the fruit hormones needed to provide protection against these outside infections. By building the mucilaginous substance, the fruit hormones work to seal off the body with all-natural means and offer a "protective hormone envelope" against bacterial invasions.

Simple Hormone Food Program Helps Heal "Stubborn Allergies"

In one reported treatment,[1] stone fruits formed the simple yet highly hormone-effective food program that healed patients and helped them recover from "stubborn allergies," which included chronic colds, internal sensitivities, and bronchial disorders. The hormones that came from fresh, raw stone fruits offered these allergy-healing benefits:

1. Fruit hormone foods helped to build up allergy fighters or antibodies in the bloodstream.
2. Fruit hormone foods neutralized toxins in the blood; that is, they helped build a natural immunity to infectious diseases and bacterial poisons.
3. Fruit hormone foods were important for the healing of wounds, the prevention of hemorrhaging, and *the building of a barrier against germ invasion.*

---

[1] *Archives of Pediatrics,* (4:52), W.J. McCormick, M.D.

4. Fruit hormone foods nourished and invigorated the white blood corpuscles and built more healthful corpuscles in the bone marrow. These white corpuscles then acted as detoxifiers in the system, devouring and casting off those bacterial agents which contributed to allergic distress. Hormones helped promote this rhythmic and all-natural process of internal cleansing.

5. Fruit hormones are especially rich in three essential amino acids—*lysine, tryptophan, and methionine,* which work to build blood health and simultaneously help fight off antibodies in the bloodstream, easing allergic ill health. In combination with the hormones, these amino acids help create a "clean sweep" in the bloodstream and pave the way for improved health, free from allergies.

Recovery Through Fruit Hormones: A simple stone fruit program, together with a "back to nature" health regimen, reportedly was helpful in hormone healing for allergic disorders ranging from the common cold to chronic and severe bronchitis!

Special Tip: In selecting fresh stone fruits, try to obtain those that are organically grown without the use of pesticides. Above all, the stone fruit should be tree or vine ripened. It should not have been prematurely picked or artificially ripened because this is a flavor loss and a hormone depletion. When stone fruits are naturally ripened, nature metabolizes the starch into a form of sugar, improving the hormone content, making the luscious fruit more soft and juicy. Nature will also help boost the nutrient supply if the fruit is left to tree- or vine-ripen by itself. Always select naturally ripened fruit.

Avoid Seedless or Stone-Free Fruits. These are fruits which have been cross-bred to reproduce without any pits or stones. These seedless or stone-free fruits (without any stones) are usually chemically fertilized with a compound which causes them to grow quickly, without seeds, by means of an unnaturally speeded up ripening process. This is contrary to the laws of nature, which hold that plants should naturally produce seeds—even those which reproduce themselves by some other method.

The stone of the fruit contains the vital part of the plant, locked up forces that enable this tiny group of cells to produce life-giving plant hormones, aided by some warmth and moisture. The stone helps the fruit grow into a plant, a bush, or a tree, bearing the rich produce—the source of fruit hormones.

To obtain a good supply of plant hormones, select wholesome fruits with their nature-created stones, pits, and seeds. These are prime sources of those hormones which serve to rebuild, remake, and recreate your biological glandular clocks, enabling them to issue forth a rhythmic supply of allergy-fighting hormones.

When stone fruits are deliciously used, together with the basic all-natural programs of glandular rejuvenation through natural living, there is hope for hormone healing of allergies, ranging from the common cold to severe bronchial disorders.

Important Chapter Subjects

1. Tree-ripened stone fruits have a rich supply of "plant hormones" that help ease allergic distress.

2. Stone fruits offer "speedy" hormones through nature-created, pre-digested, levulose-rich hormones.

3. Ralph J.'s simple fruit hormone program eased his asthmatic symptoms, when he followed a natural health program as well.

4. Stone fruit hormones offer five allergy-easing benefits.

5. Fruit hormones healed problems of chills, fever, and head cold for Barbara J.

6. George T. used a natural food program with stone fruit hormones to build resistance to chronic dust allergy.

7. Fruit hormones set up biological gland clocks in hormone rhythm to feature programmed relief while you work and sleep! A 24-hour programmed hormone supply through stone fruits.

8. Just seven easy steps help fruit hormones nourish body glands.

9. Simple reported fruit hormone food program helped heal "stubborn allergies."

10

How a Salt- and Sugar-Free Program Helps Rejuvenate the Glands' Hormone Production and Lower High Blood Pressure

High blood pressure—hypertension—is not regarded as a disease but a symptom of a disturbance within the body's endocrine gland system. A specific cause is often traced to an excessive amount of salt and sugar in the diet that alerts and over-stimulates the adrenal, pituitary, and thyroid glands. Since all of the body's glands work in harmony, one irregularity will influence the entire network, and this may lead to such symptoms as high blood pressure, nervous tension, jittery nerves, chronic worry, temperamental behavior, headaches, insomnia, and related disorders. The glands become chronically over-active, and when hormones keep gushing forth in a continual state of emergency, the body processes are unhealthy. The neurotic reaction of the over-active glands may cause the person to go from one extreme to the other. There may be days of extreme agitation followed by days of extreme lethargy and fatigue. These are the penalties to be paid by over-working the glands with an excessive amount of salt and sugar.

Seven Gland-Soothing Benefits of a Salt- Sugar-Free Program

To enable your glands to establish a natural bio-balance of body ecology and to help stabilize the functions of your hormones, you would do well to soothe your endocrines with a salt- sugar-free program. Here are seven special gland-soothing benefits to your glands as a result of such a program that will be outlined later in this chapter:

1. *Relaxed Glands Promote Acid-Alkaline Balance.* The glands issue hormones that control the formation of hydrochloric acid in the digestive system, promoting a youthful power of metabolism. Elimination of salt-sugar enables your digestive glands to make healthful amounts of hydrochloric acid, rather than be forced to use the ingested sodium chloride as part of the stomach discharge. Relax your glands so they can issue forth a healthful and natural amount of acid-alkaline hormones to help boost youthful digestion.

2. *Relaxed Glands Rejuvenate Body and Nerve Cells.* Too much salt or sugar tends to over-stimulate the glands and interfere with the absorption and utilization of food. Salt-laden hormones may also irritate delicate membranes throughout the body, causing a burn or sting, much as salt burns or stings an open wound or the eyes. Elimination of salt-sugar additives helps the gland maintain the hormone osmotic pressure of cells and tissues throughout the body. This will help maintain a healthful level of body fluids at a normal level, helping to bring about rejuvenation of the body and nerve cells.

3. *Soothed Glands Cause Natural Metabolism of Accumulated Body Fluids.* Every gram of salt will bind and hold some 70 grams of water. Every gram of sugar will cause an internal combustion action that may "burn" away valuable youth-building cells and tissues. An accumulation of body fluid may be seen as one of the contributing causes of many illnesses. To soothe your glands and enable them to issue hormones that cause natural metabolism of accumulated body fluids, and to wash and repair cells and tissues, eliminate salt-sugar from your food program.

4. *Help Your Glands Metabolize Needed Body Minerals.* The pituitary and adrenal glands work with other body glands to help metabolize calcium and phosphorus, among other minerals, as a means of healing internal inflammation, to make strong bones and also enable the thyroid to metabolize iodine. Often, if the glands are subjected to salt-sugar saturation, their metabolizing powers are weakened and the minerals are improperly processed. Help your glands issue forth valuable mineral-distributing hormones by eliminating excess salt and sugar from your food plan.

5. *Processed Salt-Sugar Products Interfere with Glandular*

Rhythm. Packaged and processed foods that contain salt and sugar may cause interference in the endocrine glandular rhythm. These packaged products contain chemicals which are unhealthy for the glands. By changing to all-natural and salt- sugar-free foods, you will help your glands become properly adjusted, and help keep them free from excessive chemical interference

6. *Healthy Hormones Promote Internal Cleansing Action.* When the glands are free from salt-sugar contamination, they are able to send forth healthy hormones that work to create "ion exchange resins," which help combat the accumulation of fluid. These same "hormone resins" are able to remove salt from the body, promote internal cleansing, and soothe the corrosive action of the burning residues left by ingested sugars. A healthful and natural hormone food program will then enable the glands to form healing hormone resins to promote this internal washing benefit.

7. *Reduce Gland Bacteria Contamination on a Salt- Sugar-Free Program.* Refined salt and sugar introduces irritating bacteria into the body and on the glands. The startled glands must work feverishly to metabolize and slough off the bacteria. They do this by issuing forth an excessive amount of hormones, which are also saturated with the infectious bacterial wastes. Since hormones pour directly into the bloodstream, the bacteria find their way to all body parts, resulting in a variety of unhealthy reactions, especially that of extreme nervousness or hypertension. To help ease this health threat, the food program should be free from added salt-sugar intake.

Your endocrine glands are precision timed to help promote youthful hormones. Any disturbance of this delicate intra-cellular balance by salt-sugar and artificial substances is incompatible with youthful health. To help improve your glandular adjustment, find the *underlying cause* of hormone dysrhythm, correct it through healthful living practices, and enjoy a relaxed and youthful body ecology.

A Sugar-Free Program Helps Boost Youthful Metabolism

Refined sugar as found in packaged and processed foods, as well as from the sugar bowl, is upsetting to the delicate gland function of calcium-phosphorus balance. Furthermore, sugar disturbs the adrenal-pituitary-thyroid rhythm and also causes the pancreas to secrete an abnormally high amount of its hormone (insulin). Much of the condition of diabetes is traced to an improper and unhealthy metabolism of the various body glands, especially the pancreas. Sugar is the culprit, causing this erratic upheaval. Elimination of refined· sugar is the first step in adjusting the biological clock glands and helping to boost youthful and healthful hormone metabolism.

How to Feed Your Glands Without Salting Them to a Nervous Hypertension

You can satisfy your taste buds and also maintain glandular rhythm with natural herbs and spices, available in specialty food shops as well as health food stores.

Hormone Healthy Seasonings: Suggested natural herbs and natural spices include bay leaf, green pepper, sage, marjoram, onion, thyme, paprika, bay leaf, oregano, lemon juice, parsley, dill seed, unsalted French Dressing, mace, ginger, and basil.

Do Not Use: Packaged products which list "salt" as an ingredient. Look for the words *salt, sodium,* or the symbol for *sodium, Na,* when you are shopping for any packaged, canned, or frozen food. If the package has no information as to how many milligrams of sodium are in the product, it is not for you. Put it back on the shelf and look for more wholesome and natural foods in a non-processed state.

NOTE: You should also pass up any items with labels listing monosodium glutamate, sodium propionate, or any other sodium compound.

Select Sodium-Free Baking Powder Products. The leavening agents of packaged bread and cake products, such as baking powder, baking soda, and sodium bicarbonate, are very high in salt. It is suggested you select salt-free baked goods made with *yeast.*

HOW TO MAKE YOUR OWN SODIUM-FREE BAKING POW-DER. If you do your own baking and prefer to use baking powder instead of yeast, you may have the following *sodium-free baking powder* prepared by your herbal pharmacist or do it yourself:

potassium bicarbonate	39.8 grams
cornstarch	28.0 grams
tartaric acid	7.5 grams
potassium bitartrate	56.1 grams

This makes about four ounces of sodium-free baking powder. Use one and a half teaspoons of it in place of one teaspoon of regular baking powder (the amount will vary at high altitudes). Add this sodium-free baking powder toward the end of the mixing time, and avoid beating too much.

How to Sweeten Your Glands to Promote Relaxed Hormone Harmony

You can help sweeten your taste buds and satisfy your sweet tooth with natural hormone food sweets.

Hormone Harmony Sweets: Suggested natural sweeteners include blackstrap molasses, honey, carob powder, date powder, rose hips powder, berry juices, fruit juices, anise seed, almond extract, cinnamon, cloves, ginger, maple juice, mint, vanilla extract, and natural tapioca. Many of these products are sold at specialty health food shops.

Do Not Use: Any packaged product or dessert which nearly always contains sugar. These include canned, packaged, frozen, pre-cooked, or freeze-dried products in any form. *Read the label.* If it says sugar, pass it up. Select wholesome and natural foods which are free from sugar additives. Pass up candy, cake, cookies, pastries, sweet rolls, or any baked goods which have been made with sugar. Select natural, whole grain foods that are baked *without* sugar. *NOTE:* Avoid any product containing "dextrose," which is the chemical name for sugar.

HOW TO MAKE YOUR OWN SUGARLESS ICE CREAM. A treat for your sweet tooth is this *Sugarless Ice Cream Delight.* Here's how to make it:

Into a glass baking dish, pour equal amounts of freshly squeezed or unsweetened pineapple juice and milk. Stir together. Place in the freezing compartment of your refrigerator. Throughout the day, stir thoroughly. When firm, you may add sun-dried fruits such as dates, raisins, figs, to further titillate your sweet taste buds. Eat this *Sugarless Ice Cream Delight* as a snack or as a dessert.

How to Help Establish a Gland-Adjusting Sodium-Potassium Balance

Earl O. was more than just the victim of hypertension and nervous glands. He had nerve-wracking insomnia, a short temper, and burst into nervous outbreaks. He was a terror to live with. He lost many customers on his laundry route, because he would rave and rant upon the slightest provocation. He was so nervous, that his blood pressure soared to a dangerous high. At times, he was so jittery, his hands would tremble when writing out an order blank, and his fingers could scarcely hold a pencil.

Correction of Sodium-Potassium Balance Eased Hypertension. Earl O.'s problem was more than just excessive salt-sugar intake. It was the maladjustment of his gland clocks and a disruption of the very delicate sodium-potassium balance. It was this imbalance that led to his nervous reactions. An excessive retention to sodium and water had led to arterial stiffening; the heart found it more difficult to pump blood through the system, resulting in Earl's increasing hypertension.

Natural Fruit Program Helps Adjust Glandular Balance. Earl O. was put on a salt- and sugar-free program and then told to eat lots of fresh fruits that were programmed by nature to have a low-sodium, yet high-potassium ratio. Nature has created these foods to contain such a built-in balance. This helped adjust the sodium-saturated glands and helped slough off the excess stored-up sodium in the system. Soon, Earl's pituitary-adrenals-thyroid were rhythmically pouring forth hormones that worked in harmony with the delicate sodium-potassium balance. The suggested low-sodium, high-potassium fruits are: raw apples, apricots, blackberries, cantaloupe, dates, figs, grapefruit, oranges, prunes, raisins, strawberries, tangerines, and watermelon.

Suggested Gland-Soothing Vegetables. Nature has also programmed the low-sodium and high-potassium balance in vegetables. Earl O. ate these vegetables as a means of helping his glands become soothed and relaxed: broccoli, Brussels sprouts, cauliflower, dry lentils, white and sweet potatoes, pumpkin, and squash.

ONE-DAY FAST FURTHER IMPROVED EARL'S DELICATE HORMONAL BALANCE. On occasion, Earl O. would go on a one-day fast—he would eat *only* the preceding lists of delicately timed sodium-potassium fruits and vegetables. For example, Earl would have a breakfast of the selected, listed fruits. Mid-morning, he would drink a fresh juice made of those fruits. Luncheon, Earl O. would have a vegetable meal of the listed vegetables. Mid-afternoon, he would drink a fresh juice made of those vegetables. Dinner, Earl O. would have either a fruit or a vegetable meal. Nightcap would consist of a glass of soothing, fresh vegetable juice.

Results: The healthful fruits and vegetables were able to work without the interference of other foods during this one-day fast; they were taken up by the pituitary-adrenals-thyroid-pancreas and other glands, metabolized, used for internal cleansing, and helped to establish a more soothing and tranquil sodium-potassium balance.

When Earl O. went off this natural hormone food program and would imbibe salt or sugar foods, his hypertension returned and his headaches became pounding sensations until he had to take to his bed. But when he followed a return to an all-natural corrective hormone food program, eliminating artificial or added salt and sugar, he was able to enjoy a good night of sleep, he had an even temper, he was pleasant to his family, friends, and customers. His hands were steady. He felt the sweet joy of hormone harmony! By self-adjusting the sodium-potassium balance, he enabled his glands to work smoothly and efficiently to maintain a rhythmic river of relaxing hormones!

The Rice Fast: Oriental Secret of Freedom from Nervous Tension

The "rice diet" has always received a lot of publicity as a means of reducing hypertension. The Oriental secret of the rice diet is that rice has almost *no* salt, and thereby is soothing to the network of glands that control the hormone-regulating blood pressure. The Orientals are known for having little hypertension because of their low-sugar and low-salt eating customs. Rice has helped further improve their glandular systems because it is one of the few "almost perfect" foods. Because rice lacks several of the essential amino acids and some other nutrients, it is not to be considered a total food. But because it is so salt-free, it is healthfully used by the glands as a means of creating a rich and powerful supply of hormones that work to metabolize corrosive wastes in the system and help expel them from the body. A one-day "rice fast" may help adjust your biological gland clocks, enabling them to dispose of excess salt-sugar through the hormones and pep up your system to enjoy freedom from tension.

HOW ALICE P. USED A "RICE FAST" TO RELAX HER GLANDS TO HORMONE HARMONY. Alice P. was subjected to everyday pressures as a private secretary for a high executive in a large firm; she was the busy mother of three during the evenings and also an active clubwoman. Because of her hectic schedule, she had to rely upon convenience and pre-packaged foods. These were so saturated with salt and sugar, that her glandular system had to work "overtime" in a frantic effort to help metabolize these additives. This created an irregular hormone reaction that made her feel pounding headaches (a typical symptom of hypertension), chronic fatigue, a nervous temperament, pounding heart, profuse perspiration, and jittery reflexes. Her punished glands reacted against the artificial foods and her hormones were unevenly distributed, creating internal disharmony. A friendly co-worker suggested she look to improvement of her less-than-healthy food plans.

Simple "Rice Fast" Brings Glandular Readjustment. The co-worker was a Yoga devotee. Her instructor, an Oriental, suggested a "rice fast" at least twice a month, as a means of helping to re-establish a harmonious hormone rhythm. The Oriental said this was a common practice amongst the more modern and affluent Orientals who now would eat processed and convenience foods, the taint of modern civilization. The Oriental instructor said that many folks come back feeling "rejuvenated" through "forever young, forever sparkling" hormones, after a rice fast. The co-worker suggested that Alice P. try this Oriental gland-soothing program.

Alice P. was desperate, so she tried the rice fast. She selected *wholesome, non-processed, natural brown rice,* which was rich in the B-complex and other vitamins, along with minerals needed to feed the glands.

Simple Program: In the morning, a bowl of boiled brown rice. In the afternoon, a bowl of baked brown rice. In the evening, a bowl of boiled brown rice in herb-flavored water. Nothing else!

Benefits: The overworked glands were treated to a rest for the day by being spared further unnecessary salt- or sugar-processed foods. With the nutrients in the brown rice, the glands (the pituitary, adrenals, thyroid, and pancreas, notably) were able to become sufficiently nourished to metabolize and cast off excessive salt-sugar wastes. When these unnatural additives were thus disposed of by the oxygen-carrying blood cells, empowered by hormone action, then Alice's hypertension eased. Just one day of this hormone food, and her nerves felt better.

Improvements Noted: Her headaches eased, her fatigue melted, her nerves felt stronger, her heart and reflexes were smooth, and she no longer perspired excessively. When the biological gland clocks had been adjusted and no longer needed to work "furiously overtime" with excess salt-sugar, her smooth rivers of hormones promoted tranquility.

What the "Rice Fast" Will Do to Soothe Your Nervous Glands

When you follow the traditional Oriental nerve-healing "rice fast" in conjunction with other outlined natural health programs, your nervous glands will enjoy these soothing benefits:

1. *Protein Feeds Your Glands.* Some eight essential amino acids in natural brown rice will nourish your glands to create healing hormones that promote relaxation and a rhythmic blood pressure. The amino-acid-enriched hormones enter into the blood and lymph, soothe the heart and lungs, relax the respiratory system, and soothe the brain and nervous system.

2. *Vitamins and Minerals Improve Hormone Health.* Rice offers thiamine, riboflavin, and niacin, along with calcium, iron, phosphorus, and potassium. The glands take up these nutrients and metabolize them for the hormones. The hormones then use these substances from whole grain, natural brown rice to nourish the skin and blood vessels, create a satisfying heartbeat, stabilize blood pressure, and maintain internal water balance. All converge to regulate the nervous glands.

3. *Rapid Assimilation by Glands.* Rice is 98% digestible, a factor that makes it rapidly assimilated by the glands. Rice starch is different and unique because it is 100% amylopectin—the most rapidly and completely digested grain starch. Once the glands assimilate this nutrient, it is taken up by the hormones to help create a soothing tranquility for the heart, blood vessels, and general nervous system.

4. *Helps Establish Glandular Adjustment.* Brown rice is non-allergenic and also has a very low fiber content, making it easy for the glands to absorb and become adjusted to. Since it is especially free of salt, it is well suited for the glands in order to issue forth "clean and sparkling" hormones that soothe rather than irritate the nervous system!

Simple—Yet Soothingly Effective. The Orientals have always regarded rice as a "food of youth." Today, we know that you are as youthful as your glands, and rice may well be the "hormone youth food" that helps ease tensions and makes you feel good all over! It is simple to go on a one-day "rice fast" to help cleanse the tensed glands. Yet, it has been reportedly effective for thousands of years and should be part of the program to help boost health while regulating the glands to promote freedom from nervous tension.

BANANAS: THE EVERYDAY FRUIT THAT EASES NERVOUS GLANDS. When nervous, try to reach for a banana! Here is an everyday food that is welcomed by the glands. The banana is very low in sodium and fat and contains no cholesterol. The secret behind its gland-feeding ability is in its unique fat (0.2 per cent or less). This fat is valuable to the glands because it has a high percentage of the three unsaturated essential fatty acids that are taken up by the glands and used to "lubricate" the nerve network, promoting a hormone-healing relaxation. The three unsaturated essential fatty acids (linoleic, linolenic, and arachidonic) become food for the glands, transformed into a salt-washing hormone flow that eases nervous tension. Though a simple and everyday fruit, the banana is a valuable gland-feeding food which helps ease nervous tension.

BANANA-RICE PROGRAM EASES GLANDULAR UNREST. In one reported study[1], bananas were used extensively to maintain glandular health in a group of some 32 hypertensive patients on a strict banana-rice program. *The Program:* Daily, the tense patients ate 1/2 pound of rice, cooked in salt-free water and served with fresh fruits and fruit juices. This fruit-rice hormone food program was effective in stabilizing glandular unrest, promoting a healing hormone rhythm, and controlling blood pressure in 20 out of 32 patients. Benefits were noted within six weeks after following this program.

A healthful rice and fruit program controls the consumption of fatty foods. This enables the hormones to work without the corrosive action of excess fat, salt, and sugar. A free-flowing set of hormones now join with the bloodstream to improve the arterial situation and help ease the conditions which may predispose the body to nervous tension. The use of rice has been known for thousands of years and is slowly coming into its own in our modern lives. Fruit, too, has been known as a hormone healer, even in the days before hormones were identified. In combination, they are the "secrets" of the past, nourishing and improving the glands to help create glandular adjustment and rhythmic hormones: the keys to relaxation.

FEED MINERALS TO YOUR GLANDS TO ENJOY HORMONE RELAXATION. Calcium, phosphorus, and potassium are just a few of the minerals to be fed to your pituitary and adrenal glands to help

---

[1] *Southern Medical Journal,* Vol. 40, Page 721, M.E. Flipse, M.D. and M.J. Flipse, M.D.

them provide hormones of relaxation. When salt-sugar from processed foods are eliminated, these minerals work to help the glands pour forth a rhythmic supply of hormones.

Oxygen, enzymes, and Vitamin C, all combine to become food for your glands, invigorated by the presence of minerals which transform these substances into materials that will provide healthful and soothing hormones.

Control Lactic Acid: An excess of white sugar from artificial sources causes an increase of lactic acid, a product of glucose metabolism and the reason behind much biochemical tension. By eliminating sugar from the food program, the tension-causing lactic acid supply is controlled; anxiety is thus eased. Replace white sugar with fresh vegetables and their juices, to furnish minerals that will help control lactic acid and also help create a healing supply of nourishing minerals. Your hormones need these minerals and other nutrients to help promote relaxation. The hormones enable the minerals to combine with lactate (lactic acid) around the sensitive endings of the nerves, preventing the acid (from sugar) from provoking nervous symptoms. Feed minerals to your hormones to give them this "buffering action" against hypertension! Help your hormones become a "shield" around raw nerves, insulating them from abrasive lactic acid. Above all, ease up and eliminate excess salt-sugar from your hormone food health program. This will help soothe your glands, improve your hormones, and promote a healthful relaxation of hypertension.

Main Points in Review

1. To help control hypertension, go easy on the salt-sugar shakers, and ease up on packaged foods that have been salt-sugar treated.

2. Your glands reap seven basic benefits when you follow a salt-sugar-free eating program.

3. Relax your glands by following a simple salt- sugar-free program.

4. Sweeten your glands the natural way to promote relaxed hormone harmony.

5. Help establish a gland-adjusting sodium-potassium balance.

6. A one-day "fruit fast" and a one-day "rice fast" helps establish hormone harmony and relaxation of tense nerves.

7. Earl O. and Alice P. enjoyed freedom from hypertension through hormone harmony.

8. Banana-rice programs eased tensions by correcting glandular unrest.

9. Minerals control lactic acid formation, a source of glandular torture. Ease this torment with fresh vegetables and their juices and a salt- sugar-free eating program.

11

The Raw Hormone Food Plan to Help Rejuvenate Glandular Production of "Feel Young" Hormones

Fresh, raw fruits and vegetables as well as whole grains are storehouses of substances that feed the endocrine glandular network system, to help rejuvenate the "feel young" hormones. Within these fresh, raw hormone foods nature has placed *living* substances, such as vitamins, minerals, and enzymes, that are used by the glands for the creation of energetic and youth-building hormones. To help feed your glands these living substances, your food program should consist of natural, fresh, raw fruits and vegetables as well as whole grains.

How Hormone Foods Help Glands Promote Youthful Digestion. The living substances in uncooked raw hormone foods are taken up by the endocrine glands to help promote "feel young" hormones for youthful digestion and create these two essential benefits:

1. The thyroid, parathyroids, and adrenals use living substances to bring about youthful metabolism and an assimilation of carbohydrate, fat, protein, and minerals. These metabolized substances are then transformed into such youth-building hormones as thyroxine, parathormone, cortin (the hormone complex, including cortisone, which helps resist against arthritic-like stiffness), epinephrine, and adrenalin substances. Once these enriched hormones are sent pouring into the bloodstream, they help to promote a youthful digestion and

131

assimilation and alert a healthful physical energy, heart action, and cheerful nervous system. The endocrine glands obtain these "hormone foods" from the *living* vitamins, minerals, and enzymes in raw foods.

2. The endocrine network needs the living substances in raw foods to help provide an alkaline reserve to equal the acids which are in large supply in the blood and tissues. In raw foods, the substances are used by the pituitary and thyroid to influence the adrenals to issue forth those hormones that help maintain digestive equilibrium. Once hormones have bathed and washed the internal organs with their living supply of digestive nutrients, especially enzymes, there is an improvement in the acid-alkaline balance, and a more youthful digestive-assimilation rhythmic pattern.

Sources of Raw Foods for Youthful Hormones: Fresh, raw, uncooked fruits, vegetables, seeds, nuts, and grains are rich in nature's own hormones. These are absorbed by the endocrine glands, which prepare them in a manner to be taken up by the body's hormones and help adjust a *youthful* hormone rhythm. *Suggestion:* Eat fresh foods raw if they can be eaten without cooking. Cook *only* those foods which *must* be cooked.

How Raw Foods Enable Hormones to Promote Internal Scrubbing

Fresh, raw fruits and many vegetables are needed by the endocrines in order to extract those substances which are used by hormones to promote "internal scrubbing." The adrenal and thyroid hormones metabolize these raw foods, gathering up the bulk which they impart, via the hormones, to the residues, thereby giving the muscular mechanism of the intestine an opportunity to be effective in helping to move the residual mass. This hormone action enters into the process of washing and elimination. *The hormones use the fiber of the raw foods to give the digestive organs their daily scrubbing.*

"Feel Young" Hormones Help Rejuvenate the Bloodstream. The endocrine glands take up the nutrients in raw foods, extract their disease-fighting substances, and "feed" them to the hormones. The enriched hormones then use these substances to enrich the quality of the bloodstream—in particular, the "feel young" hormones help nurture and create white corpuscles, which are needed to help fight ravages of illness and aging. *Raw foods* offer these elements to the

hormones, to help nourish the bloodstream with youthful disease-fighting white corpuscles. The endocrine glands are better nourished with uncooked foods.

HOW A RAW FOOD BREAKFAST HELPED NOURISH "AROUND THE CLOCK" YOUTHFUL HORMONES. Joyce E. would feel a recurring numbness in her hands and fingers, just several hours after she began her day as a statistical typist. There were times when the long columns of figures on the sheet would swim in her head and become confusing, even though she knew there was nothing wrong with her eyesight. Added to her distress was a perpetual "tired feeling" and the "knot" that became tighter and tighter in the region between her shoulder blades. There were times when Joyce E. would have a gnarled, twisting sensation if she would try to straighten up after bending over her typewriter for a brief time. Even at home, Joyce E. would experience a wrenching twist when straightening up, following some dusting or vacuuming chores in the living room. She refused to believe it was old age creeping up on her. She decided to adjust her basic living patterns to "natural" living standards.

Follows Glandular Adjustment Program. She emphasized more natural, wholesome foods, obtained sufficient sleep at night, and would go for frequent walks to help limber up. These natural health programs did relax the stiffness and helped promote a more youthful hormone rhythm. But she still experienced premature tiredness and chronic fatigue. She now went on a simple and delicious *raw food breakfast* plan as follows:

Raw Fruit. Seasonal, fresh, raw fruit began the breakfast. The vitamins, minerals, and enzymes in the raw fruit were eagerly taken up by the endocrine glands for the manufacture of healthful, self-scrubbing hormones.

Whole Grain Breakfast Food. A bowl of natural whole grains available at most health stores and organic food outlets followed the fruit course. *Example:* Hulled sesame seeds, millet flakes, and hulled sunflower seeds in a bowl of slightly warmed water or slightly simmered milk. *Benefit:* The slightly simmered water or milk creates a gland-pleasing action known as *hydrolysis.* This action creates a gentle pre-digestion of the vitamins, minerals, enzymes, and amino acids in the whole grain, helping to soften the cellular structure of that grain. Eaten in this manner, the pre-digested food helps release nutrients, making them more readily available for the glands to prepare them to be used by the hormones. The "hormones" of the grains are then speedily released to the body's own hormone rivers to help promote youthful health.

Benefits of a Seed Milk Beverage. By whirring two heaping tablespoons of any organic seed (alfalfa, wheat, oats, beans, sesame, fennel) powder with one cup of water in a blender, Joyce E. fed her endocrine glands with a drink of a rich supply of *living* hormones.. *Benefits:* The Seed Milk Beverage has as much as 36 per cent protein of an *alkaline* type, which makes it soothing to the glands. The hormones then become healthfully alkaline to help boost a youthful digestive power. Seed Milk also has a natural oil which is rich in those unsaturated fatty substances needed to *lubricate* the glandular machinery and create a free-flowing hormone supply. This helps perk up the body processes and makes the glandular clocks tick forth in rhythmic balance.

WHY JOYCE E. FEELS YOUNG AGAIN. The special Raw Food Breakfast Plan was more than just tastefully delicious. It was food for the glands, promoting healthful hormones, alerting the nerve responses, regulating the rate of metabolism, balancing the use of phosphorus and calcium (minerals needed to promote hormone harmony and tranquility), and helping muscular efficiency through a nourished adrenal glands process. Joyce E. found that she could now read up and down a long column of statistical figures without seeing the numbers swim around. Furthermore, when the healthful raw food breakfast was able to regulate the blood pressure, maintain water balance, and build resistance to stresses through stimulating the medulla (segment of the adrenals) to issue forth healthful adrenalin, Joyce E. felt a gradual relaxing of the tight "knot" between her shoulder blades. She began to "unwind"—thanks to the living substances in her "Seed Milk Beverage" that nourished her endocrine glandular system.

Follows Raw Hormone Food Program for Healthful Hormones. Joyce E. now followed the gland-feeding raw hormone food program. Daily, she would eat a fresh, raw fruit salad for lunch. She would eat a large raw vegetable salad before her dinner in the evenings. At times, she would eat a seasonal raw salad as a complete meal in itself. *Benefit:* the hormones in the living foods are then metabolized without interference of other substances from *cooked foods.* It was this occasional "raw food fast" that helped promote healthful glands and youthful hormones. Joyce E. now felt "young all over," thanks to rejuvenated and well-nourished hormones.

How Raw Vegetables are Nature's "Hormone Youth" Factories

Fresh, raw vegetables are nature's prime sources of those ingredients that are known to be "hormone youth factories" or *enzymes*. Cooking will destroy these internal "hormone fountains," so it is healthful to your glands if they are fed with raw vegetables. In effect, *your endocrine glands drink from the "hormone fountains" in the raw vegetables.* The gushing fountains are sources of youth-building enzymes.

How Glands Are Rejuvenated by Hormone Enzyme "Fountains." The endocrine glands drink of these "hormone fountains" in raw vegetables. They are able to perform their rhythmic biochemical, biophysiological, and biopathological actions and reactions because of these enzymes, which serve to regulate and control the processes of living organisms. The glands take up the enzymes from the raw vegetables, use these enzymes to bring about such internal actions as metabolism, building and rebuilding of billions of body tissues and cells, purifying the bloodstream, helping in assimilation of nutrients, and nourishing the entire system of body organs. Your endocrine glands need these enzymatic "hormone fountains" in raw vegetables.

Enzymatic hormones are intimately connected with virtually all of the gland-causing healing and regenerative methods. They aid in digestive functions and participate in assimilation and elimination. The glands use these enzymatic hormones to *break down complex foods* into simple *living* substances which can then be poured directly into the bloodstream. Enzymes are able to perform these youth-building benefits without themselves becoming involved in the change. For this reason, they are called catalysts.

Each Enzymatic Hormone Has an Individual Benefit. Of the more than 700 different enzymatic hormones in the system, each one has its *individual* benefit. One enzyme activates production of insulin by the pancreas gland. Another enzyme promotes digestion of starch when the food is properly salivated and chewed. Another enzyme will metabolize sugars and starches to be stored in the liver. Each gland needs the family of enzymes to help promote a rhythmic production of *youth-building* hormones. The absence or the *weakening* of any enzymatic hormone causes a basic slowdown of the entire inter-connected glandular network. This makes it essential to provide the system with "hormone fountains" of enzymes found in fresh, raw vegetables.

HOW VEGETABLE HORMONE FOODS TURNED BACK THE "AGING CLOCK" FOR NORMAN. Norman B. was an "eat and run" type. He was "all business." As a buyer for a large department store, he was under constant pressure, had to meet schedules, and was constantly "on the go." This disturbed his eating patterns, not to mention his basic health programs. He rarely ate raw foods. He preferred "instant foods" or those that were pre-cooked and required little eating effort or time. The constant emotional-physical strain, together with nutritional inadequacies, played havoc with his glandular system. His biological clocks began to run down. His hormones were sluggish. His basic health declined. Norman B. looked haggard and worn out.

Co-Worker Suggests Vegetable Hormone Program. His co-worker had undergone endocrine therapy and was familiar with an all-natural way, through my books, to help nourish the glands to produce rhythmic rivers of hormones. He suggested that Norman B. try a "raw vegetable fast" program—just raw vegetables throughout the day. *Benefits:* The depleted glands could use their sluggish powers to work solely upon the vegetables, extract their hormones, become better fed, and help send forth a stream of youth-building hormones throughout the body. Without interference from other foods, the body's glands then devote maximum time to raw vegetables and are able to become enzymatically enriched from nature's own hormones. It was a simple, yet highly rejuvenating program that Norman B. followed. Note the following benefits.

Five Ways in Which Vegetable Hormones Promote Glandular Rejuvenation

Fresh, raw vegetables offer a supply of nature's hormones to help promote *glandular rejuvenation* in these five basic ways:

1. *Soothing, Natural Hormone Tonic.* Raw vegetables with all-natural hormones are soothing to the glandular system and provide a balanced supply of nourishment for the endocrine glands. *Vegetable hormones* are nature created and serve to complement the sluggish or deficient supply in the system, without over-working or over-taxing the tired glands.

2. *Vegetable Hormones Offer Stress-Shield Protection.* The all-natural hormones in vegetables are used by the glands to encircle and shield the millions of blood, bone, and body cells and body tissues—a protection against the stresses and tensions of unhealthful daily

living. They coax the adrenals with a natural gentleness until these glands issue forth healing cortin and adrenalin to help build resistance to external stimuli, such as stress, heat, cold, and toxic invasions. Vegetable hormones offer this natural internal shield protection.

3. *Vegetable Hormone Foods Replenish Aging Cells and Tissues.* To help bolster the weakening effects of tired glands, such as the pituitary and pancreas, as well as the parathyroids, the vegetable hormones are *natural supplements.* They work to create those substances that remake aging and broken down cells and tissues. If the body's own hormones are insufficient, these cells and tissues may break down, predisposing to premature aging. Therefore, nature has created "enzymatic hormones" in vegetables to become a natural and healing supplement, assist the sluggish glands, and nourish them to full health. These vegetable hormones help promote cellular sustenance and nourishment to help turn back the aging clock.

4. *Vegetable Hormone Foods Promote Youthful Assimilation.* The vegetable hormones perform a valuable function in helping to "lubricate" the digestive tissues and arterial networks. In so doing, they help boost youthful assimilation. This is often regarded as the key to helping turn back the aging clock. A youthful assimilation is beneficial in that it enables the living substances from foods to enter into the making and remaking of body tissues and organs. Vegetable hormones help "soften" and "lubricate" the organs involved with digestion and enter into the enzymatic rhythm of youthful assimilation.

5. *Vegetable Hormones Are Quickly Absorbed by Glands.* Because nature has created these all-natural hormones, she has made them speedily assimilable by the glands. It is this intrinsic power that makes vegetable hormones so beneficial—within an hour after eating a plate of raw vegetables, the hormones are sent into the bloodstream to help perform the youth-rebuilding factors and health restoration benefits.

Norman B. Feels Young Again After Vegetable Hormones Turned Back the "Aging Clock." The rich supply of natural enzymatic hormones from raw vegetables did help Norman's glandular health. When he would devote just *one day a week* to raw vegetables, his biological gland clocks were healthfully adjusted; his hormones were precision timed and were sent ticking-ticking-ticking throughout his body to promote healing of distress symptoms. He had actually reversed the "aging clock" through vegetable hormones!

How to Eat Raw Foods to Feed Your Glands
with Nature's Hormones

1. Serve all fruits raw, whenever possible. (Cooking of fruits or vegetables will inactivate enzymatic hormones and deplete other essential hormone-feeding substances.)

2. Eat most vegetables raw. Serve several different raw vegetables at one time to offer different vegetable hormones and a variety of taste.

3. Serve your raw foods *first.* A unique benefit is that the enzymatic hormones are more effective when introduced to the glands *before* other foods are ingested to create any weakening of their function. *Begin* a meal with raw fruits or vegetables to help provide a fresh supply of enzymatic hormones to the glands for their nourishment and youthful regeneration processes.

4. Fresh, raw vegetables with *raw cashews or nuts* and raw seeds add up to a *harmonious* enzymatic balance that offers a healthful "rhythm" to the biological gland clocks. In this combination, there is a supply of vitamins, minerals, enzymes, and proteins, all taken up by the glands for creation of healthful hormones to promote youthful processes.

5. Boost the power of vegetable hormones by adding nutritional yeast (Brewer's Yeast flakes, available at most health food stores) to your raw vegetable salad. *Benefit:* The nutritional yeast flakes are prime sources of those amino acids that go into the biological creation of internal hormones. This offers "hormones plus" power to the natural vegetable hormones in a raw salad. It provides a prophylactic benefit when the body needs healing hormones from nature.

ADDITIONAL SUGGESTIONS: Help your family and yourself become adjusted to eating more raw foods. When you plan meals, include more and more raw salads. Fruits should be eaten raw. Vegetables, too, should be eaten raw, except those that are distasteful and need some steaming. Occasionally, go on a "raw food" fasting program. Devote an entire day to raw foods through this simple-easy-effective plan: *Breakfast:* Fresh, raw fruit bowl with seeds and nuts. Seed or nut milk. *Luncheon:* Fresh, raw vegetable salad with Brewer's Yeast, powdered seeds, and whole grains. Vegetable juice. *Dinner:* Large bowl of fresh, raw vegetables with whole grains. Seed or nut milk.

In addition to their healthful hormone-feeding benefits, raw foods offer a glandular revitalizing reaction on the vital body organs. At many beauty farms and rejuvenating health clinics, raw foods are used regularly to help alert the endocrine glandular network, to cause the glands to gush forth their "youthifying" properties, and to build new tissues, new health, and new youth—through natural hormones!

Practical Points to Remember

1. Raw foods help promote "feel young" hormones for youthful digestion by creating two essential benefits.

2. Fresh, raw foods enable hormones to promote internal scrubbing.

3. A simply prepared, raw food breakfast offered Joyce E. a powerhouse of "around the clock" youthful hormones.

4. Fresh, raw vegetables are nature's "hormone youth" factories.

5. Glands are rejuvenated by raw food hormone enzymes.

6. Note the five ways in which vegetable hormones promote glandular rejuvenation.

7. Follow the unique, five-step raw hormone food program to feed your glands with nature's hormones.

12

How Natural Hormone Foods Help Women Feel "Forever Feminine" After 40

The youthfully feminine appearance of women is controlled largely by their hormones. Actually, women undergo regular changes throughout their lives, sparked by the ebb and flow of their female hormones. In particular, some time between their late 30's and their mid 50's, their hormones undergo distinctive changes with the result that their bodies become influenced by these glandular variations. The female sex glands (the ovaries) slow down their production of estrogen and progesterone. With the gradual cessation of these two hormones, women's bodies begin to react to distinctive symptoms.

A decline in production of these hormones may bring about such symptoms as nervous tension, brittle and porous bones, and a susceptibility to arthritis, high blood pressure, and cardiovascular disorders. Many women are able to go through this "change of life" or menopause with minor discomforts. But many more find themselves growing flabby, with pads of fat accumulated on hips and thighs and dry, loose, wrinkled skin. It is this so-called "loss" of femininity that calls for corrective food programs to help the body's glands make up for their hormone decline.

HOW HORMONE FOODS HELP NOURISH SLUGGISH GLANDS. Nutrients in natural and non-processed foods will be taken up by the pituitary gland, to be sent, via the bloodstream, to the ovaries, to help them supplement the decline of progesterone

140

hormone. Natural food hormones soothe the ovaries and influence the thyroid and pituitary glands, which are largely responsible for the health of the female glands. These natural food hormones further influence the sympathetic nervous system and help adjust the blood vessel rhythm to ease the symptoms during this trying time in the female's middle years. Natural food hormones may be regarded as a form of nature's own estrogen supplementation. The nutrients in wholesome foods are able to help adjust the biological gland clocks so they can provide an all-natural, substitute nourishment for the sluggish ovaries.

NATURAL HEALTH PROGRAMS IMPROVE HORMONE BALANCE. Natural health programs build an internal "hormone fountain" to ease the disruption and erratic behavior of the post-40 ovarian function. While both *estrogen* and *progesterone* are essential in helping to keep a woman "forever feminine," these hormones work in harmony with those produced by the adrenal glands and by conversion of other steroids in the liver. While estrogen production is slowed up, the body continues to have its own self-produced supply, sparked by natural health programs. It remains to the food hormones to help supplement the diminishing supply from the ovaries.

Natural Hormones Require a Healthy Body Through Natural Hormone Foods. In order for the natural food hormones in the corrective food programs outlined herein to be of benefit, it is essential for the entire body to be properly adjusted in a healthful rhythm. Since the body's network of glands are so precision adjusted and so inter-related, it is necessary for *all* of them to work in healthful harmony. If the internal organs are healthy and the neuro-endocrine system healthfully nourished, in the natural menopause, the intake of natural food hormones is soothing and gradual, so that the pituitary and other glands can take up the slack and the woman is able to enjoy a "forever feminine" feeling with the joy of living. Your glands are as healthy as your *entire* body. Use natural healing programs for the *whole* body and enjoy the benefits of a healthful hormone rhythm, even when the ovaries undergo normal changes.

THE MINERAL THAT ACTS AS A BONE-BUILDING HORMONE. During the decline of estrogen hormone, the problem of osteoporosis or demineralized, fragile bones may occur. A decline in the flow of estrogen hormone leads to a negative balance of calcium and phosphorus. *Furthermore, the osteoblastic (bone-building) cells are under direct estrogen control. The more estrogen, the more osteoblastic activity.* The more estrogen, the stronger the bones and the less there is of a risk of fragile bones or osteoporosis.

The Simple Mineral Food to Boost Hormone Strengthening of Bones. A simple mineral food is that of bone meal—available in capsule as well as powder form at most health stores. Bone meal is a powerhouse of calcium and phosphorus as well as the other minerals, including magnesium, which is taken up by the pituitary gland, properly metabolized, and then poured directly into the bloodstream. These minerals are then used by the endocrine network to help supplement the declining estrogen flow; the minerals work to become absorbed into the structure of the bones, to ease the problem of brittleness. In actuality, the pituitary and adrenal glands are "hungry" for calcium and phosphorus and the other minerals in bone meal, from which they make a natural estrogen hormone substitute to help make up for the body's own decline.

How Barbara G. Used Minerals to Ease Her Hormone Starvation. Barbara G. knew that she was approaching her "change of life" when she experienced heart palpitations, recurring headaches, and an unceasing sense of anxiety. Most significant was her low back pain—one of the earliest symptoms of a declining estrogen supply and "hormone starvation" in the body's bones. She followed a more natural health program, but emphasized mineral supplementation, specifically that of bone meal. Here is what Barbara G. did to help her glands adjust to the changes with adequate estrogen-making minerals:

FOREVER FEMININE MINERAL TONIC. Three times daily, Barbara G. would prepare an all-natural Forever Feminine Mineral Tonic by using this simple recipe:

> 4 tablespoons bone meal powder
> 4 tablespoons cod liver oil
> 1 glass of raw vegetable juice

Stirred vigorously, this was a treasure of calcium, phosphorus, magnesium, and vitamins, as well as proteins.

Barbara G. would drink this Forever Feminine Mineral Tonic three times daily. *Benefits:* The Vitamin D in the cod liver oil worked as a catalyst (expediter) in permitting the calcium's speedy absorption into the structure of the bones. The pituitary-adrenal glands needed the Vitamin D as an "energizer" to help metabolize the calcium and send it streaming through the hormone rivers and to nourish and strengthen the osteoblastic (bone-building) cells. It was a task that was ordinarily performed by the estrogen hormone, but since Barbara's ovaries underwent a normal decline in the production of this hormone during her middle years, she used the Forever Feminine Mineral Tonic as a natural hormone substitute.

THE B-COMPLEX HORMONE BROTH FOR NERVE HEALTH. Since all the glands and nerves are under the tension of readjustment during the middle years, there is the need for the B-complex family of vitamins to help put this jangling orchestra into more soothing tune. Barbara G. would prepare this easy broth, a powerhouse of the valuable B-complex vitamins:

    4 tablespoons Brewer's Yeast flakes
    2 tablespoons desiccated liver powder
    1/2 teaspoon kelp
    1 glass tomato juice

Stirred vigorously, this B-Complex Hormone Broth would be taken at least twice daily by Barbara G. *Benefits:* The supply of thiamine, riboflavin, pyridoxine, niacin, and pantothenic acid, working with the valuable calcium, phosphorus, potassium, magnesium, and iron, as well as the more than 16 all-natural amino acids, were taken up by the pituitary-adrenal glands and then combined with the sluggish estrogen hormone, acting as a hormone booster tonic! Barbara G. found that when her endocrine glands were thus invigorated by this hormone food, her symptoms of nervous unrest, insomnia, heart palpitations, perspiration, and hot-cold reactions (flashes), were all greatly eased and less discomforting. The powerhouse of all-natural nutrients in the B-Complex Hormone Broth helped a sluggish and declining estrogen supply become supplemented with natural hormones.

UNIQUE BENEFIT OF BREWER'S YEAST. Brewer's yeast is a *food.* Many regard it as a natural and healthful gland food. When it is taken up by the glands, its released nutrients then work to help make up for a declining estrogen supply. But Brewer's Yeast is regarded basically as a *hormone food* for the endocrine glands.

Results: Barbara G. found that through a wholesome and natural hormone food program that was high in protein, modest in carbohydrates, reasonable in fats, and the elimination of refined foods (elimination of sugar and salt), and a wholesome return to nature, together with the use of the Forever Feminine Mineral Tonic and the B-Complex Hormone Broth, she was able to meet the approaching "change" with youthful confidence. She looked and felt youthfully feminine. She began to rely on her *natural* hormones, taken through *natural* hormone foods!

How Cold-Pressed Seed Oils Act as Natural Hormones

Substances in cold-pressed seed oils are able to help make up for the decline in production of the body's own hormones. The tormenting symptoms of the "change" may be eased when the starved endocrines are given valuable nutrients that act as natural hormones, to help make up the deficiency of the declining activity of the ovaries.

Seed Oils Boost Blood Health. Estrogen is needed by the bloodstream to help nourish and replace the red cells in the bone marrow. During the female "change," a decline of estrogen often leads to a depletion of red blood cells, a premature disintegration in the bloodstream; the bone marrow cannot replace the cells fast enough and the result is a form of anemia. To help provide a natural estrogen hormone activity, seed oils are especially valuable to the woman who wants to improve her bloodstream and thereby increase her youthfulness.

How Seed Oils Act as Blood-Building Estrogen. The pituitary-adrenal glands take up Vitamin E and the unsaturated fatty acids in seed oil, using them to help supplement the weakening estrogen, which joins with iron to form hemoglobin-rich blood cells. The hormone-like ingredients in seed oils act to enrich the bloodstream and nourish the sponge-like interior of the bone marrow in which youth-giving red cells are made. Seed oils may well be regarded as natural hormones which act in place of the declining estrogen.

Seed Oils Help Prolong Youth. The youth of a woman is often equated with the availability of her estrogen supply. When there is a diminishing supply, there may be visible reactions of declining youth in the form of cracked and wrinkled skin, thinner hair, cold hands and feet, nervous unrest, susceptibility to infection, and premature tiredness. Nature has put substances, including Vitamin E, in seed oils to create an all-natural, estrogen-acting benefit. Nature has endowed seeds and their cold-pressed oils with those substances that help prolong youth, *acting as an all-natural estrogen supplement.*

Special Hormone Benefit: Substances in seed oils work as healing hormones to meet the challenge of fragile red cells. An estrogen deficiency may lead to a "low" plasma Vitamin E level and a susceptibility of red cells to hemolysis (breakdown) by hydrogen peroxide in the bloodstream. A prolonged estrogen deficiency leads to extreme fragility of the red cells and their destruction by hydrogen peroxide. Seed oils, when metabolized by the endocrines, are valuable for their Vitamin E and unsaturated fatty acid content; the glands send these substances throughout the bloodstream and enrich the health of the red cells, helping them maintain integrity and improvement. In effect, the seed oil hormones perform a natural anti-oxidant function in the body—protect the cells by preventing the formation of hydrogen peroxide which destroys those cells.

The hormones in seed oils strengthen the outer membrane of the red cells, reducing the risk of more frequent ruptures and the spilling of hemoglobin. The hormones in seed oils offer intra-cellular enzymes needed for membrane integrity. While estrogen normally helps in this process, a deficiency may render the bloodstream susceptible to breakdown that is seen in the premature aging of women over 40 who go through the "change."

KINDS OF SEED OILS: Select *cold-pressed* seed oils at most health stores and natural food outlets. You have a choice of such hormone-feeding seed oils as: almond oil, apricot kernel oil, oil of avocado, cod liver oil, corn oil, cottonseed oil, olive oil, peanut oil, rice bran oil, safflower seed oil, sesame seed oil, soy oil, sunflower seed oil, English walnut oil, and wheat germ oil. Use them singly or in combination, when preparing a salad, when using any type of oil at all.

VITAMIN E: THE NATURAL HORMONE TONIC. In a reported study[1], a physician told of being able to replace or supplement a declining estrogen hormone supply, and helping to ease the emotional and physical symptoms of the "change" by an all-natural method—giving Vitamin E, regarded as a Natural Hormone Tonic.

Benefits of Natural Hormone Supplementation: Vitamin E reportedly helped to stabilize the blood pressure, supplement the deficiency of estrogen, and dilate the smaller blood vessels so that the nervous concentration of blood in the abdomen became relieved. When the glands absorbed Vitamin E, their issuing hormones soothed the body-heat-regulating mechanism so as to reduce nervous sweating, and with it, the relaxation of the sympathetic nervous system.

Reported Cases: The physician reported treating 35 women with hormonal decline symptoms, over a three-month span. He gave each woman 100 International Units of Vitamin E, daily. The doctor reports that the natural hormone supplement offered relief to more

---

[1]Henry A. Gozan, M.D., *New York State Journal of Medicine,* May, 1952.

than half of the women. By means of supplementation with Vitamin E, the natural hormones promoted a feeling of well-being, eased the nervous tensions, and helped to keep the women looking and feeling more youthful.

Apparently, Vitamin E helped regulate a hormone balance, helped maintain calcium in the bones, and promoted a better rhythm of the biological body glands.

How Jean E. Used Natural Hormones to Adjust Gland Clocks. Jean E. had seen her older sisters and close relatives go through the "change" with nerve-wracking symptoms. She had seen her eldest sister develop severe cardiovascular disorders, not to mention migraine headaches as well as severe depression during the "change." The eldest sister never fully recovered and she was prematurely old in her middle 40's. Jean E. prepared herself in advance for the change. This was wise. She reasoned it would help nature if she would use natural hormones in her early 30's so that she could just adjust her gland clocks so they would tick away in soothing rhythm, even after she reached her 40's and 50's. Here is her simple and all-natural program:

1. *Healthful Hormone Foods.* Jean E. gradually eased up and eliminated her artificial and synthetic foods and replaced them with healthful, natural hormone foods. She preferred fresh fruits and vegetables, fresh meats, fish, eggs, and whole grain breads. She eliminated processed foods, which were chemically saturated and sugar- salt-drenched, because these additives upset her delicate, precision-timed hormone balance.

2. *Nightly Rest.* To meet the challenges of the internal changes, she obtained a healthful night's rest. She would avoid upsetting situations, steer clear of nervous stimulations, and aim for peace and relaxation. This put her in tune with her body harmony.

3. *Natural Hormones from Foods.* Jean E. increased her natural hormone food intake. She would boost her vitamin and mineral intake, increase her intake of seed oils, and use fresh fruits and vegetables that were eaten raw, whenever possible. In particular, she boosted her Vitamin E intake occasionally through Vitamin E supplement capsules. This helped create a natural hormone feeling to meet the challenge of the ovaries' decline in estrogens and progesterone.

4. *Adequate Exercise.* A dwindling estrogen level often tempts a woman into inactivity. Jean E. was wise in knowing that lack of

physical activity and immobility not only leads to overweight, but also causes a further decline in hormonal activity. She would take daily walks, occasionally go on a hiking trip into the country with her friends, and even joined a local supervised physical fitness club. By keeping her body active, she was able to alert her endocrine networks and keep them functioning properly, so that even when there was a decline in estrogen, she met the challenge by keeping in good physical condition, together with natural hormones.

Adjusted Gland Clocks Keep Her "Forever Feminine." By keeping her body healthfully nourished and properly taken care of, by following natural health programs, Jean E. was able to maintain the production of non-ovarian estrogen at a satisfactory level. Even after her body's ovaries' activity ceased entirely, she had built up a so-called reserve with natural health programs and was able to cooperate with her adrenal-pituitary glands, adjusting them so that she was "forever feminine" through natural hormones.

FRESH FRUITS AND VEGETABLES OFFER NATURAL HORMONES. Nature has put vitamins in fresh fruits and vegetables that are able to help promote a hormone easing of menopausal-type leg cramps. A decline in ovarian-produced estrogen often leads to weakness in the walls of the capillaries, which are the tiniest of the blood vessels.

Many women over 40 experience leg cramps, which may be traced to a shortage of oxygen in the muscles because of poor functioning of the capillaries supplying those muscles. This is a symptom of a decline of estrogen, produced by the body's glands.

To help meet this challenge, the woman should turn to fresh fruits and vegetables. Hormone-like agents in these natural hormone foods are the bioflavonoids, hesperidin, rutin, ascorbic acid, and other substances. These help the body improve its oxygen supply, aid in promoting capillary strengthening, enrich the blood vessels, and improve the cushioning of the deep vascular bed beneath the skin. Ordinarily, the bloodstream carries estrogen and other hormones to these regions, to promote resistance to leg cramps and frequent bruises. But when the ovaries show a decline, it is nature's signal to help supplement the decrease with natural hormones in fresh fruits and vegetables.

Benefits: Fresh, raw fruits and vegetables have a good supply of hormone-like bioflavonoids, among other ingredients, which are taken up by the glandular system to perform a healing of broken capillaries. They further work to keep needed oxygen in the blood for an extended period of time to strengthen the arteries and capillaries. These hormone-like bioflavonoids further act as a natural estrogen supplement, picking up the slack and working in harmony with the rest of the glands to help readjust and correct the biological clocks that determine femininity and youthfulness at all ages.

The arrival of the 40's in a person's life is a new and encouraging era of life. Cooperate with nature, help the hormone changes with natural hormone foods, help correct the biological gland clocks to face the wonderful years ahead—with health and happiness.

In Review

1. The "change of life" is a natural process; the key to unlock the mystery of declining ovarian hormones is in natural food hormones. A healthy body can issue forth healthy hormones to meet the responsibilities of the "change."

2. Nature health programs help supplement dwindling supplies of estrogen and progesterone.

3. A simple mineral food helps boost hormone-strengthening bones.

4. Barbara G. was helped by a Forever Feminine Mineral Tonic. She helped correct maladjustments with natural programs and the B-Complex Hormone Broth.

5. Cold-pressed seed oils act as natural hormones.

6. Vitamin E is regarded as a natural hormone tonic.

7. Jean E. eased through the "change of life" with a natural, four-step health program. Fresh fruits and vegetables offer hormone-like benefits.

13

How Protein Hormone Foods Help Keep the Male Glands Young and Healthy

Natural "protein hormones" from healthful foods are needed by the testes and prostate gland for an overall feeling of youth, virility, and health. These protein hormones are sources of youthful nourishment for the male glands, the two sources of fertility, virility, and a "forever young" feeling of energy. The testes secrete a hormone known as testosterone, which affects secondary sex characteristics in the male and keeps him sexually fertile and virile. The prostate gland secretes a clear fluid-like hormone that contains substances that nourish the fragile microscopic cells whose health is essential for youthful vigor. Chief among the substances in the prostatic fluid is the youth-building protein.

The testes and prostate gland are able to provide protein to their respective hormones from the foods that are eaten. Protein, together with an adequate supply of unsaturated fatty acids, work in harmony to nourish the prostate and testes and enter into the manufacture of male hormones. These same hormones are as youthfully healthy and as body-mind stimulating as the available supply of protein. If there is a deficiency of protein, then the malnourished testes and prostate gland will issue a weakened supply of male hormones. The biological gland clocks become maladjusted and the evidences of premature male aging may then occur. It is healthfully beneficial to nourish the testes and prostate gland with "protein hormones" to help create protein-rich male hormones. These, in turn, help keep the male feeling young in body and mind.

149

A combination of unsaturated fatty acids with natural protein work to nourish the cells and tissues of the prostate gland (located just below the bladder and encircling the urethra from which it exits via the bladder). The 40-plus male who has an increasing need to get up nightly for bathroom trips, or has an unnatural feeling of "fullness" in the bladder region, would do well to correct his program for better daily living. He needs to eat healthfully nourishing hormone foods, obtain adequate rest, and feed protein to his prostate gland—all of which will keep it from enlarging.

How Seed Sprouts Help Enrich the Hormone-Making Testes and Prostate Gland

Truly, "living foods" are seed sprouts. Sprouting is also a fast way of improving the nutritional value of food. Seeds are tiny storehouses in which nature has hidden the procreative powers that make possible the continuation of life. Without the sprouting ability of seeds, life would end. In the tiny seed sprout, there is a treasure of hormone-making elements that are valuable to the testes and prostate gland.

Protein Source in Seed Sprouts. Seed sprouts are prime sources of protein as well as unsaturated fatty acids in a nature-created combination that helps boost the health of the male glands, especially the prostate. The protein in seed sprouts has been likened unto its own seed hormones. These same seed hormone elements aid in nourishing the prostate gland, help boost its hormone-making powers, and improve basic health.

Five Male Gland Benefits of Sprouts. Here are some of the benefits to your male glands as made available in seed sprouts:

1. Sprouted seeds become rich sources of Vitamin C. The healthy B-complex and E vitamins are also increased during the sprouting process.

2. The cellulose in the seeds is softened so that the sprouts may be eaten raw and easily assimilated for use by the testes and prostate gland.

3. Sprouting reduces the starch content of the seeds to more simple carbohydrates, increasing ease of digestion and speeding assimilation into the hormones.

4. Seed sprouting helps ease the sometimes disagreeable gas-generating problem of beans, at least for some people.

5. Sprouting breaks down the seed protein into its component amino acids, helping in digestion and hormone assimilation of the seed protein.

Unique Benefit: During sprouting, the seeds passed the test which is used to determine the completeness of a hormone food—*they sustained life all through the reproductive cycle for several generations.* The same nourishment in these seeds helps invigorate the prostate gland, which can then send forth better youth-building hormones. Seed sprouts may well be the most essential source of "protein hormones" for the male "youth gland" that is his prostate.

SELECTED SEEDS FOR SPROUTING. Obtain *organic* and *untreated* seeds for sprouting from an organic farm. (Many commercial seeds are treated with fungicides such as mercury; this can be disruptive to the delicate glandular system.) High-protein seeds include lentils, alfalfa, red clover, radish, peas, Mung beans, oats, sunflower, pumpkin, wheat, and rye. *TIP:* Both wheat and rye seeds must be cleaned carefully so that there are no broken seeds. These will not sprout but will ferment. NOTE: Use any organically grown seed that will grow. It should be fresh and whole and of the highest quality.

10 Easy Steps to Sprout Seeds in Your Own Kitchen

Use the back of your kitchen cooking range because there is comfortable warmth in that location. Be sure it is not too hot to prevent germination. Other locations in your apartment or house may also be selected for a comfortable warm spot. Here are the 10 easy steps:

1. Select clean, fresh, untreated, unbroken seeds. Freshness is important.
2. Discard all but the clean, whole seeds.
3. Wash and drain seeds and place in a sprouter—you may use a two-quart jar.
4. Cover seeds to four times their volume with lukewarm water, overnight.
5. Pour off the water in the morning. Wash and rinse the seeds thoroughly, pouring off the last water.
6. Cover the open end of the container with cheese cloth. Tie securely.

7. Now invert the jar and place in a dark location, tipped slightly.

8. About every three hours, place the jar under the running cold water of your kitchen tap and rinse thoroughly.

9. When the sprouts are about 2 inches long, they're ready to use.

10. Rinse well. Wash in water to float the hulls. Skin off the hulls and drain sprouts. Refrigerate in plastic bags. Try to use within two or three days. You will be feeding yourself a powerhouse of protein hormones in a nature-nourished combination with unsaturated fatty acids. These hormone foods work in rhythmic harmony to nourish the testes and prostate gland, to help enrich a healthfully young supply of virile hormones for the male.

HOW TO EAT SEED SPROUTS. They are best when eaten raw. But this need not be the rule. Alfalfa seed sprouts are tasty when eaten plain or sprinkled over salads or used in soups. Wheat sprouts may be eaten raw as a relish or placed in salads. Red clover sprouts are palatable as a salad or in soups. Radish, lentils, peas, Mung beans, and other seed sprouts may be used for munching, combined with a chopped raw salad, as part of a healthful vegetable sandwich, or sprinkled over a whole grain breakfast cereal. All sprouts go well with any tossed salad, fruit or vegetable. They are excellent in cottage cheese. *Gourmet Tip:* Use sprouts in sandwiches in place of lettuce.

HOW TO DRINK YOUR SEED SPROUTS. Combine sprouts with any juice (or milk) and put in the liquefier-mixer. Blended together, no one suspects he is getting a *Seed Sprout Drink*, it is so flavor-packed and tastefully nourished.

THE JAPANESE HORMONE FOOD SECRET FOR NEW YOUTH. An ailing accountant, Ralph N., had to go to Hawaii for his health. While the warm climate and fresh air made Ralph feel better, he still was prematurely aged and felt much older than his 44 years. His Japanese cook was well in his 60's and quite popular with the ladies! What was his secret? The Japanese said that Tokyo Bean Sprouts are the staple of the diet of his countrymen. The amazing virility of Japanese men in their 60's, 70's, and 80's may well be based upon the powerhouse of potent protein in Tokyo Bean Sprouts. The cook prepared whole batches of Tokyo Bean Sprouts for Ralph N. by following this simple plan:

TOKYO BEAN SPROUTS. Cover the bottom of a Pyrex or other glass dish with one layer of soybeans. Cover with lukewarm water. Soak overnight. Next morning, pour off water. Cover dish. Place in a corner. Next morning, add fresh water and rinse off all excess. The sprouts will appear on the third day. They are tender enough to eat on the fourth day.

Secret Gland Benefit: Raw soybean sprouts are an amazing source of delicately balanced protein, unsaturated fatty acids, and Vitamin C that comprise the same fluid found in male hormones! Throughout Japan and the Orient, raw bean sprouts are looked upon as an aphrodisiac. This may well be the secret of Japanese virility—Tokyo Bean Sprouts, with their powerhouse of hormone-making nutrients.

Results: Ralph N. ate a bowl of such freshly prepared Tokyo Bean Sprouts almost daily. He recovered sufficiently to be able to look and feel better.

How Unsaturated Fatty Acids Helped Rejuvenate the Prostate Gland

In a reported case program[1], 19 men who had disorders of their prostate gland, were able to feel rejuvenation by improvement in their eating programs. In particular, these 19 men were put on a natural hormone food program. All foods were wholesome, non-processed, and prepared in simple yet glandularly soothing manners. The emphasis was on natural hormone foods, together with the use of unsaturated fatty acids.

Benefit: Protein in wholesome foods as well as the unsaturated fatty acids promoted an androgen-hormonal influence to produce regenerative, invigorating, and youthfully vitalizing influences on the endocrine glands, especially the testes. These influences further stimulated an invigorating supply of youth-building male hormones in the prostate gland.

Results: Nearly all of the men experienced a "rejuvenation" as well as a reported *glandular regeneration.* The prostate gland was healed. The so-called "aging" was reversed as the men further experienced an increase of sexual libido, better strength in their limbs, and general improvement in physical and mental well-being, all due to the hormone food program.

Gland-Feeding Oils: The gland-feeding unsaturated fatty acids are found in cold-pressed oils, such as almond oil, avocado oil, corn oil, cottonseed oil, olive oil, peanut oil, rice bran oil, safflower seed oil, sesame seed oil, soy oil, sunflower seed oil, and wheat germ oil.

[1]J.P. Hart, Sc.D. and W.L. Cooper, M.D., "Vitamin F in the Treatment of Prostatic Hypertrophy," Report No. 1, Lee Foundation for Nutritional Research, Milwaukee, Wisconsin.

Select natural oils that are cold-pressed and free from preservatives, such as those sold by most health food stores and organic food outlets.

10 Ways to Feed "Complete Protein Hormones" to Your Male Glands

The male glands will benefit when being fed what is known as "complete protein hormones." Some proteins contain all the known building blocks required for the construction of glandular tissue and the manufacture of youthful hormones. Some other proteins contain only a portion of the so-called "essential amino acids," and the glands are thus given only a portion of youth-building nourishment.

When you eat protein, your enzymatic hormones must split it into these *amino acids* to get them through the membrane walls of your male glands. Proteins, as such, are not diffusible. It is up to the enzymatic hormones to break them down into these amino acids, which can then be used by the prostate and other male glands for the making of youth-restoring hormones. To help give your glands most of the "essential amino acids," to create a rhythm within your biological clocks, here are 10 examples of nearly complete amino acid patterns:

1. Raw vegetable greens in a salad plus raw cashews or other raw nuts.

2. A raw vegetable drink made with raw nuts or seeds or seed sprouts.

3. Raw green vegetables with mashed avocado dressing.

4. Sprouted seeds plus a raw green salad.

5. Large green salad plus Swiss or Cheddar cheese chunks.

6. Large green salad plus natural cottage cheese with wheat germ.

7. Large green salad plus sesame seed oil or any seed oil for dressing.

8. Raw green vegetable salad with a raw egg mayonnaise or health store mayonnaise.

9. Raw green vegetable salad plus yogurt for a dressing.

10. Raw green vegetable salad with any lightly cooked meat, fish, or egg. (*Unique Benefit*: These protein foods will be more readily digested because the raw salad will supply the amino acids that might otherwise be destroyed by the heat of the cooking of the meat, fish, or egg.)

Suggestion: Twice daily, eat two of the different numbered items listed above as a means of helping to create "complete protein hormones" in an amino acid balance for your glandular network.

How Erwin T. Helps Keep His Male Glands in Youthful Activity

Although he is over 40, Erwin T. is able to keep his prostate gland in working harmony with the rest of his endocrines, including the testes, by following an easy yet highly effective "rejuvenation" program. Quite simply, here is Erwin T.'s program:

Natural Hormone Foods. He eats fresh raw fruits and vegetables daily. He avoids processed, packaged, or canned foods, especially those containing white sugar and/or white flour. He soothes his glands with whole grain breads and cereals.

Protein Booster. Daily, Erwin T. eats a handful of freshly sprouted seeds to help feed his glands with valuable youth-building protein hormones.

Hormone Cocktail. Twice daily, Erwin T. makes a tasty yet hormone-feeding cocktail by adding four tablespoons of cold-pressed seed oil to one glass of freshly prepared raw vegetable juice. He adds four tablespoons of any available nut powder. (Pulverize organic nuts on a seed mill or merely run through a blender until a powder is formed.) Erwin T. mixes these three all-natural foods together with his blender or just a spoon. He drinks this Hormone Cocktail by imbibing one glassful at noon and another glass in the early evening.

Benefits: The unique combination of complete amino acids, together with the unsaturated fatty acids, as well as the vitamins, minerals, and enzymes, all work together in a special rhythmic harmony. They work in this combination to help invigorate the endocrine gland clocks to feed amino acids (digested protein) to the testes and prostate gland. The resulting youthful hormones that then flow in natural rhythm are enriched with these natural nutrients, promoting a feeling of youth and health in body and mind.

Delicious Vegetable Combination as Hormone-Booster. Erwin T. has found that *two ordinary vegetables,* when served together, provide a good amino acid balance. These two vegetables are: corn and sweet potatoes. When served in a *combination,* they offer all the essential amino acids for the hormone-making prostate gland.

Special Gland-Nourishing Combination. Nuts, seeds, and whole grains should be eaten in *combination* with raw, green, leafy vegetables. *Benefit:* They combine metabolically to provide a complete amino acid pattern that is well utilized by the glands to then create youth-building hormones. Erwin T. has discovered this *combination* and he will eat, daily, a salad comprised of nuts, seeds, and whole grains, together with seasonal *raw* vegetables. It is this simple, yet highly effective combination that has enabled his male glands to work in harmonious rhythm, ticking off a steady and balanced supply of youth-building hormones.

Today, Erwin T. may well be on the threshold of so-called "middle age," yet his above-outlined, all-natural, and amazingly easy-to-follow program, has helped him look and feel younger. Rather, his well-nourished glands have given him "forever young" hormones!

The Meatless Source of Protein Hormones— The Case of Edward S.

Edward S. found that meat disagreed with him. He preferred living as a vegetarian. In his middle years, he ran the risk of a protein deficiency. Yet, he was able to boost his protein supply by eating whole grains, seeds, lentils, and nuts. In particular, *soybeans* gave Edward S. a good source of meatless protein hormones.

Meatless Protein Program: Edward S. increased his soybean eating program. This gave him the essential amino acids needed by his testes and prostate gland to keep functioning healthfully. It might be added that heretofore, Edward S. was troubled with having to get up several times during the night for bathroom trips; he looked pale and wan. His energy capacity was somewhat reduced and he would walk with a stooped gait. (He was all of 48!)

Brewer's Yeast Protein Potion. Edward S. would mix four heaping tablespoons of Brewer's Yeast in one glass of tomato juice. Stirred vigorously, he would drink this in between his meals. This unique combination gave his male glands a healthful supply of such hormone-making amino acids as histidine, isoleucine, lysine, methionine, phenylalanine, threonine, tryptophan, and valine. But most important, the Brewer's Yeast Protein Potion gave Edward S. an *amino acid balance* that could then be more biologically absorbed into the prostate, to help boost the supply and quality of his hormones. Brewer's Yeast, the all-natural hormone food, could thus offer "complete protein" in a form that was absorbed by the endocrine system to promote youthful hormones.

BENEFITS: After following a high meatless protein hormone food program, Edward's endocrines, especially his prostate, responded quite favorably. He no longer needed to make unnecessary or excessive nightly bathroom trips; his complexion and energy improved; his posture was more youthful and upright.

HOW TO PLAN A MEATLESS PROTEIN PROGRAM: Daily, your hormone-feeding program should consist of soybeans, whole grains, nuts, seeds, lentils, millet, buckwheat, brown rice, raw fruits, and raw vegetables. Used in a variety of combinations, together with the aforedescribed Brewer's Yeast Protein Potion, and seed sprouts, you will be helping to feed your prostate and other male glands with a good balance of essential amino acids—from meatless foods.

Wheat Protein: One-half cup of raw wheat germ has close to 25 grams of protein, nutritionally equivalent to more than a quarter-pound of meat! *Suggestion:* sprinkle raw wheat germ over your whole grain breakfast cereal, use it in a vegetable cocktail, sprinkle it in soups, over salads, in a glass of fruit juice.

Yeast Protein: Four tablespoons of Brewer's Yeast has close to 20 grams of protein, equivalent to about a quarter-pound of meat nutritionally! *Suggestion:* Mix Brewer's Yeast in fruit or vegetable juices; sprinkle the flakes over whole grain breakfast cereal, in soups, over fruit or vegetable salads.

Nut Protein. To help provide yourself with a more complete protein pattern, eat nuts. Mix them up. Brazil nuts offer methionine while cashews offer lysine; sunflower and sesame are good sources of histidine and lysine. Mix up nuts and munch them daily, chop for a raw salad, liquefy with water in a blender for a healthful Nut Protein Shake.

Select a Variety of Foods: In helping to feed protein hormones to your glands, select a wide variety of foods. This helps provide a proper balance of amino acids. Do not confine yourself exclusively to one specific food. Do not limit yourself just to green leaves (lettuce) or roots (parsnips) or seeds (corn or wheat) or fruit (apples, peaches). Each of these foods is incomplete by itself. A *combination* of them, together with other outlined wholesome foods that have leaves, roots, tubers, seeds, fruits, and vegetables, will help give your system a more complete amino acid pattern that then becomes more beneficial and well-utilized by the endocrine glands of the body.

The prostate gland and testes are one of the biological clocks that work in rhythmic harmony with the other body glands. Protein hormones, as well as a natural and healthful plan of living, help to nourish the body's network of glands, and boost the efficiency of the prostate and testes—the male glands that may well be the key to virile youth and health.

Summary

1. The male glands need protein nourishment to help in the creation of youthfully healthy hormones.

2. Seed sprouts enrich the hormone-making testes and prostate gland. Follow the simple 10-step plan that tells you how to make sprouts right in your own kitchen.

3. How a selected number of men experienced "prostatic rejuvenation" when put on a natural food program with emphasis on unsaturated fatty acids.

4. Lubricate the prostate gland with cold-pressed seed oils.

5. To feed your male glands "complete protein hormones," try the 10 suggested examples of nearly complete amino acid hormone food patterns.

6. Erwin T. experienced glandular regeneration on a simple program of natural hormone foods, a Hormone Cocktail, and a special combination of two ordinary vegetables.

7. Edward S. was able to boost his "meatless protein" supply through special natural hormone food programs.

8. The Brewer's Yeast Protein Potion, Wheat Protein, Yeast Protein, and Nut Protein are sources of balanced amino acid patterns to feed the prostate and other male glands.

9. Select a variety of hormone foods to create rhythmic harmony between all the biological gland clocks.

14

A Natural Hormone Food Program to Help Build a Healthier Heart

The heart is the master timekeeper of the body's glandular clocks. When the heart is properly nourished, it is able to function smoothly, to adjust the various body glands so they can send forth a rhythmic supply of healing hormones. But when this master timekeeper is abused by faulty living habits, it declines in efficiency, causing an interruption in the glandular clocks, disturbing the smooth flow of youthful hormones. By using natural hormone foods, together with simple oxygen-boosting exercises, the heart is given nourishment and ventilation, which enables it to help adjust the biological glandular clocks to promote a youthful hormonal rhythm.

How Seed Oils Promote Heart-Healing Hormones

Cold-pressed oils from such sources as pumpkin seeds, sesame seeds, soybeans, squash seeds, olives, almonds, corn, cottonseed, linseed, peanut, sunflower, safflower, and other seeds and grains are prime sources of unsaturated fatty acids, as well as Vitamin E, which is needed by the heart to enable its mechanism to work with adequate nourishment and oxygen.

Unique Benefit: Seed oils contain a combination of unsaturated fatty acids, *together* with Vitamin E, that can be assimilated and digested in a form to be used by the heart to help in the creation of hormones. It is this *combination* that makes seed oils so beneficial, since Vitamin E cannot be properly assimilated without the presence of these unsaturated fatty acids. Together, they are taken up by the endocrine glandular network and sent via the bloodstream into the heart, which then becomes aerated (given oxygen) and nourished so it can continue its rhythmic pumping, which, in turn, adjusts the biological clock glands. It is all part of the harmonious teamwork of the body's organs. Seed oils may well be the "fuel" that enables the heart and endocrine glands to keep functioning in a youthful hormone rhythm.

Five Hormone-Boosting Benefits of Seed Oils

The heart is a solid muscle which must continuously pump blood to the billions of body tissue cells. The heart empowers the glandular system to pump forth its valuable supply of youth hormones. Seed oils are needed by the heart to promote a constant, ceaseless supply of oxygen and nutrition to the glands so they can then use these life-giving elements in the making of hormones. Your heart and endocrine glands work in harmony to help boost a healthful supply of hormones. They receive their vitality from seed oils, together with other programs of healthful living. In particular, cold-pressed seed oils offer these hormone-boosting benefits:

1. *Heart-Gland Homeostasis.* Seed oils carry oxygen and nutrition to the heart and the glands to create a hormonal-youth equilibrium known as *homeostasis:* a complete internal-external balance. Seed oils furnish "breathing nutrients" to the trillions of cells in the heart as well as the glands, to enable them to work in harmony to issue forth youthful hormones that are properly oxygenated and nourished. This helps create *homeostasis,* a natural blending of the heart-gland network to promote youthful hormones.

2. *Heart-Healing Hormone Foods.* Seed oils work to send refreshing hormones into the bloodstream. In the form of Vitamin E together with the unified unsaturated fatty acids, these hormones help create a natural anti-thrombin (that which reduces bloodclots) in the bloodstream. These heart-healing hormones that are nourished by Vitamin E and unsaturated fatty acids reportedly do not interfere with the normal clotting of blood in a wound, nor with the normal healing process. Instead, these hormones enable the blood to flow more smoothly, and help accelerate the healing of burns and wounds and other disorders. It is the enrichment of these hormones with

Vitamin E and unsaturated fatty acids that helps promote a heart-healing benefit.

3. *Hormones Bring Oxygen to the Heart.* The presence of Vitamin E with the unsaturated fatty acids in the hormones helps boost the youth-giving function of oxygen within the body. That is, the hormones use these seed oils to create an action of natural anti-oxidation in the body. The hormones help the bloodstream get through the heart to provide oxygen as a means of easing the threat of anoxia (lack of oxygen), which is the trigger that sets off anginal or heart pain. The hormones require oxygen to help the heart in its need for "breathing" power. The combination of Vitamin E and unsaturated fatty acids thus give the hormones their needed "heart breath."

4. *Hormone Foods Help Melt Unwanted Internal Scar Tissue.* Seed oils offer nutrients to the hormones that work to help prevent excessive scar tissue production, a forerunner of heart distress. Hormone-nourished blood will then offer healing substances to the heart to help melt unwanted scar tissue and related obstructions.

5. *Hormone Foods Help Dilate Blood Vessels.* Seed oils feed the hormones with substances that help them dilate constricted blood vessels. The hormones use these substances to help open up new pathways in the circulatory systems and ease blockages produced by clots and hardened arteries.

Cold-pressed seed oils enrich those hormones which bathe the heart muscle, nourish it, improve the bloodstream, and help the "master timekeeper" in its youth-building tasks.

How Natural Hormone Foods Help Rejuvenate the Heart

Seed oils are able to help slow up the so-called inevitable process of aging by sending a natural anti-oxidant hormone supply to the heart. This helps slow and even reverse-repair the aging processes.

The so-called aging process is initiated by an interaction between substances that cannot be eliminated because the body must have them. These include oxygen and various essential fatty acids. The glands need unsaturated fatty acids to send nutrients via the hormone-enriched bloodstream to build and rebuild the various membranes of the individual cells of the body.

These hormones enable the membranes to bind the cells, hold them together, and permit and encourage the flow of vitality and youth-giving nutrients into the cell. These hormones help the membranes in their work to permit and encourage the flow *out,* into the bloodstream, of waste substances such as carbon dioxide. The hormones need oxygen from seed oils in order to bring about this rhythmic rejuvenation. The cellular membranes depend upon the oxygen from the hormones to build and rebuild the cells of the heart and body. The main source of oxygen comes from seed oils that are used to nourish the glands and hormones that enter into the bloodstream. The key to heart rejuvenation would be to provide enough oxygen to the hormones to enable them to build the cells and tissues of the heart and body.

Hormone Food Enables the Heart to "Breathe." Seed oils offer substances to the hormones that help bring breathing air to the heart. The membranes of the cells are highly susceptible to "free radical" (cellular blocks) reactions. Denied sufficient oxygen, the membranes may swell. The cumulative total of destructive reactions caused by these free radicals may cause cellular death. The hormones become weak if they are deficient in Vitamin E, unsaturated fatty acids, and other nutrients, and are unable to help the heart resist and recover from destructive attacks. The premature aging process thus begins. A key to helping the heart and cells become "oxygenated" would be in the hormones which bring air to these vital organs. Such air comes from healthful living programs, natural foods, and, most essential, seed oils.

Hormone Foods Help Soothe Aging Heart. Seed oils send lipid anti-oxidant factors streaming into the bloodstream to be carried to the heart. These hormones then help prevent oxygen from combining with fatty acids to form peroxides and cellular blocks. By helping to eliminate the cause of the damage for much of what we know as an "aging heart," these hormones help to slow the aging process, itself. The hormones need the substances in seed oils in order to help promote the metabolic changes within the cells to soothe and rejuvenate the "aging heart."

Hormone Foods Help Maintain Heart-Glandular Balance. A properly nourished glandular system helps promote an internal balance with the heart system. Seed oils help counteract the threat of cellular deterioration and help maintain an internal metabolic balance and rhythm between the master timekeeper—the heart—and the biological gland clocks. Seed oils will help spare loss of oxygen and help enrich the hormones with their heart-rejuvenating benefits.

How an All-Natural Hormone Food Program Promoted Heart-Healing Hormone Rhythm

Jeff R. felt "winded" after having to walk up a short flight of stairs. If he had to walk several blocks, his face was flushed and he could scarcely catch his breath. He tired easily. He looked much older than his 48 years. Where he could previously go out with the boys for a bowling game twice a week, he now found it was so exerting, he was tired afte. the game had begun for only a few moments. Evenings, Jeff R. would just "flop" in a sofa chair to watch television. He had little desire to do anything else. His concerned wife had heard about heart tensions, knew that Jeff's father had succumbed to a heart attack, and she wanted him to improve his health to help ease the threat of such an illness. Here is the all-natural hormone food program recommended to her:

1. *Seed Oils Replace Hard Fats.* She would use any available cold-pressed seed oil for cooking, as a salad dressing, even as a butter substitute when preparing a sandwich made of whole grain bread. *Benefit:* Nutrients in the seed oils entered into the hormones to help oxygenate the heart, helped boost heart-blood circulation, and brought a breath of life to the internal organs.

2. *Natural Sweets Replace White Sugar Foods.* Jeff's wife replaced white sugar with organic honey, natural maple syrup, date powder, rose hips powder, and natural jam. She refused to let him eat or drink anything with white sugar. *Benefit:* White sugar drains out the B-complex vitamins from the system in order for it to be digested. This causes a hormone deficiency of the B-complex vitamins and the heart suffers from such a deprivation.

3. *Fresh Fruit and Vegetable Juices.* Jeff's wife gave him lots of fresh fruit and vegetable juices that were natural sources of Vitamin C. This vitamin is taken up by the hormones, which use it to strengthen the blood vessel walls, nourish the capillaries, and also rejuvenate the body's connective tissues. *Benefit:* The hormones then use Vitamin C to help reduce the cholesterol level in the bloodstream and melt the arterial cholesterol. The hormones would use Vitamin C as a protective buffering action in all problems of stress and tension. Jeff's entire body benefited by raw juices. The hormones used these nutrients to help in the building and rebuilding of the heart and other internal organs.

4. *Whole Grain Hormone Foods Offer More Nourishment.* Whole

grain breads, cereals, rice foods, and breakfast foods were part of Jeff's hormone enrichment program. *Benefit:* These whole grains (unrefined and natural) sent a supply of various vitamins, minerals, enzymes, and amino acids, to the glands, which used these metabolized nutrients to help maintain a healthful blood cholesterol level—the key to a youthful heart. The hormones thus "bathed" the heart muscle, sent oxygen to the circulatory system, and helped boost the feeling of youth.

5. *Smoking-Liquor-Caffeine Were Taboo.* Smoking, liquor, and caffeine-containing beverages were to be eliminated. Jeff R. was disinclined to give up these habits, but faced with the threat of an "aging heart," he slowly condescended. *Benefit:* Tobacco sends wastes into the hormones which disturb metabolism, drain out oxygen, and raise the fat level in the bloodstream. Liquor causes a burning or corrosive action on the glands and may lead to cellular destruction. Caffeine (including coffee, tea, and soft drinks) causes a glandular maelstrom. The glands must work in a frenzy to metabolize the caffeine. This takes them away from other vital functions, weakening their powers. Caffeine further blocks off iron absorption by the hormones and may also interfere with the hormone's use of inositol—a B-complex vitamin needed by the heart for youthful functioning. Incidentally, soft drinks or cola drinks have as much caffeine as the average cup of coffee, not to mention harsh artificial flavors and chemical preservatives. In Jeff's case, restriction and elimination of cola drinks further helped his hormones increase their power to send healthful rivers to the heart.

Results: It took several months of natural, healthful living, which also called for nightly rest, moderate and doctor-approved exercises and sports, mild walking, and peace and quiet, until Jeff R. felt young again. Now he could walk up several flights of stairs without getting out of breath, he was a favorite and steady player at the bowling alley, he looked young and felt so rejuvenated, that he would take out his wife almost weekly for an evening of entertainment. She deserved it. His wife had helped Jeff's glands become "heartfully young" again!

Five Simple Exercises to Alert Heart Hormones

The glands need to be exercised, just as do most of the other body organs. To help boost their hormone-making function, moderate exercise sends a stream of much-needed oxygen into the circulatory system, to be taken up by the glands which then send it to the heart, via the hormones. Here are five very simple but highly effective exercises that help send oxygen through the hormone rivers to the billions of body and.tissue cells that are in and around the heart:

1. AIRPLANE PROPELLER EXERCISE. Stand tall. Keep heels and toes together. Lift up your chest. Draw in your stomach. Keep your shoulders back, your head high. Keep your chin in. Your hands should remain relaxed at your sides. Slowly, start a circular motion forward. Your hands and arms make a complete circle forward along the sides of your body, much in the manner of a moving airplane propeller. Slowly pep up the speed until you make the circles as quickly as possible. Begin by doing one dozen circles forward. Increase by several circles a day until you can count up to 50.

2. REVERSE PROPELLER EXERCISE. Keep the same position as No. 1. Now, instead of making circles with your hands forward, make the circles backward in the opposite direction.

3. HORMONE ENERGIZER. Keep the same position as No. 1. Now, stretch out your arms and hands horizontally at shoulder height. Each hand forms a half circle as you do this exercise. Your right hand strikes your left shoulder, and your left hand strikes your your right shoulder at the same time, then alternately. Your arms are criss-crossed alternately . . . right over left, left over right . . . (repeating), while you slap your shoulders vigorously. *Note:* make it vigorous so that each time your arms are flung open back to the starting position, your chest is pushed forward. Begin by doing 10 times. Gradually work up until you can do it comfortably 25 times.

4. LEG-FOOT HORMONE VIBRATIONS. Stand tall. Keep your feet about 10 inches apart. Your arms are relaxed at your sides. Now, place all weight on your left foot. Raise your right foot off the ground about 8 inches. Make short kicks (about 5 inches) in a forward motion—as hard as possible. Your leg should be vibrated from your hips to your toes. Now, alternate by standing on your right foot and kicking with your left foot. Begin by making 10 kicks with each foot. Slowly increase the amount daily until you can kick up to 25 times or more with each foot. *Note:* Make this a vigorous motion to help promote the circulation and send healthful hormones throughout the entire body.

5. UPPER BODY CIRCULATION BOOST. Stand tall, your feet about 12 inches apart. Lean forward from your waist. Your arms

hang comfortably relaxed at your sides. Comfortably shake your head from side to side, forward to back. Begin slowly; do this exercise just a few times until your upper body becomes adjusted to this circulation booster.

Overall Hormone Benefits from Simple Exercises: Your heart is a muscle that requires exercise just as do your body glands. These· simple exercises enable the endocrine glands to become more flexible, sending forth healing hormones that will help boost circulation and flow freely through the blood vessels. These exercises help the hormones send purifying oxygen to the lungs and create an internal aeration that is refreshingly healthy and stimulating to all body organs.

Special Tip: Exercise should *train* the body . . . not strain the body!

GOLDEN OIL BONANZA TONIC. To help send a stream of oxygen-bearing nutrients into her hormones, Phyllis E. drinks this simple and delicious all-natural Golden Oil Bonanza Tonic three times daily:

> 4 tablespoons peanut oil
> 1 glass raw vegetable juice
> 1 tablespoon apple cider vinegar
> 1 tablespoon organic honey

Mix thoroughly together. Drink one glass in mid-morning, a second glass in mid-afternoon, a third glass as a nightcap. The Golden Oil Bonanza Tonic sends a treasure of nutrients, including the valuable unsaturated fatty acids, Vitamin E, and various minerals and enzymes, directly into the digestive system. Here, Phyllis E.'s digestive glands cause metabolization, later sending these nutrients to the endocrine system and hormones. The hormones then work to help protect the heart cells by preventing the formation of hydrogen peroxide. (This toxic ubstance is a known destroyer of red blood cells, initiating the chain of events that cause heart distress.)

Extra Benefits of Golden Oil Bonanza Tonic: When Phyllis' hormones received the substances in this all-natural hormone food tonic, they worked to strengthen the outer membranes of her red blood cells, easing the threat of destruction and the spilling of valuable hemoglobin. The enriched hormones then sent intra-cellular enzymes to the heart, to help promote membrane integrity. They worked to establish a heart-healing, body-strengthening mechanism, to help create a feeling of youthful vitality and energy. When Phyllis E. followed other previously described natural health plans, with natural hormone foods, adequate sleep, moderate exercise, and relaxed living habits, she was able to enjoy life with youth and vigor . . . thanks to "forever young" hormones that were nourished with seed oils and natural nutrients.

HOW TO FEED HEALTHY HORMONES FOR YOUR HEART. A corrective hormone food program calls for the use of unsaturated fats, low fat, low salt, low sugar, and a moderate amount of carbohydrates. The emphasis should be on non-processed and natural foods. In particular, use seed and nut oils from such sources as these foods: avocado, olives, pumpkins, sesame, soybeans, squash, almond, beechnut, Brazil nut, cashew nut, filbert, hazelnut, peanut, pecan, pistachio, walnut, corn, cottonseed, safflower. Increase your intake of whole grain millet, oats, natural brown rice, wheat germ, and whole grain corn. Use seed and nut oils for your salad dressing. Use seed and nut oils in your baking and cooking. You will be giving your hormones the substances they need to help feed health to your body and heart.

Checklist of Important Points

1. Replace animal fats with seed oils to help enrich your heart-healing hormones.

2. A wide variety of natural cold-pressed oils offer an adventure in culinary tastes and health benefits for the glands and heart.

3. Seed oils offer five special hormone-boosting benefits.

4. Jeff R. promoted heart-healing hormone rhythm when he followed a simple, all-natural nutritional program.

5. To help alert heart hormones, try the simple exercises in this chapter. Just a few minutes may make all the difference in health to your biological gland clocks.

6. The tasty Golden Oil Bonanza Tonic helped Phyllis feel youthful with her "oiled" glands.

7. Feed on healthy hormones for your heart by following natural health programs and using a variety of seed and nut oils in baking and eating.

15

Water Therapy for Boosting Natural Hormone Activity

"Water contains great healing power," noted Father Sebastian Kneipp, the famed Bavarian mountain healer. His successful all-natural "water cure" for alerting the glands and stimulating natural hormones, attracted thousands of people throughout the world to his healing clinic in Woerishofen, Bavaria. As the recognized pioneer of water cure, he put his patients on an all-natural food program, emphasizing bathing as a means of helping to boost sluggish glands and sleepy hormones to help promote overall mental and physical health.

Father Kneipp noted that fresh, "alive" water would provoke a natural stimulation of the skin surfaces, which sent an electrolyte reaction into the endocrine glands to help alert them to a healthful adjustment or a "winding up" of these internal clocks of youth.

According to his program, water bathing would bring youthful circulation to the endocrine glands, invigorate the bloodstream (the carrier of hormones), and help promote a rhythmic balance within the body. Once the biological gland clocks were properly adjusted by water immersion as well as liquid drinking, then the hormones could bathe the internal organs with their youth-giving elements, thereby promoting basic healing, boosting circulation for the upper parts of the body, improving the health of the bloodstream, and pepping up lazy processes.

His programs were highly successful and are in wide and increasing use in many of our modern healing institutions. Hydrotherapy (water therapy), raw juice fasting programs, special bathing programs, specially designed needle-spray showers, all form part of the healing programs to restore vigor to stiff limbs and wake up lazy glands and hormones.

Father Sebastian Kneipp was responsible for creating a new healing specialty called "koorortology," from the German word *kurort,* which means "health resort." Other European healers followed the lead in creating health resorts or health spas. Tens of thousands come to these health spas to take the Kneipp water cure to help boost the health and vitality of the body's glands. When followed in combination with the basic health laws outlined in this volume, there is new hope for rejuvenation with nature.

The Natural Hormone-Boosting Values of "Living Water"

According to Father Kneipp's program, fresh, "alive" water would help boost the hormone values by alerting the biological gland clocks in this manner: *sun-kissed water from swift-flowing lakes and streams, drenched by rainfall, enriched by sunlight, transported solar energy, biological oxygen, and beneficial micro-organisms to the skin surfaces. Here, these all-natural "energizers" worked to stimulate the skin cells, sending a magnetic reaction through the pores, to help alert-awaken sluggish glands and improve the health of the internal organs.* This adjusting of the biological gland clocks, according to Father Kneipp, was the source of all-natural hormone activity that was then healthfully sent streaming throughout the body. By using water bathing, the alerted hormones could work to promote youthful health of body and mind.

A visit to any of these "water cure" spas in Europe would show the onlooker how men and women would wade knee-deep and waist-deep in the cool, fresh streams. Many of Father Kneipp's patients would experience glandular reawakening by bathing in the natural, solar-energized waters of the creeks, rivers, and streams surrounding his Bavarian clinic. Today, the health resort has spread throughout Europe and America. Father Kneipp's water cure, as he called it, has helped many thousands upon thousands. His programs may also be followed in the home, for those who are unable to visit a health spa. Here is how water therapy may be done right in your own home.

How the Sitz Bath Soothes the Male Prostate Gland

There are three types of sitz baths that reportedly help soothe the male prostate gland, the key to his prolonged youth and vigor: warm, cold, and contrast.

1. *The Warm Sitz Bath.* Fill the tub only midway with comfortably warm water. Sit in this warm water no longer than five minutes, with your knees drawn up so that only your feet and your pelvic region are immersed in the water. *Benefit:* The water exerts a soothing effect upon the prostate gland, sending a rhythmic flow of youthful energy into the pelvic area, the source of prolonged youth. (The Europeans call this the "youth bath" because the increased circulation to the glandular centers help keep a man young.) Male patients in European spas take one such warm Sitz Bath daily.

2. *Cold Sitz Bath.* Fill the tub only midway with water that should be from 50-60 degrees. It may be as cold as you can *comfortably* endure it. Again, sit in this cold water no longer than five minutes. Your knees should be drawn up and only your feet and pelvic region should be immersed in the water. *Benefit:* The cold water creates a pleasant circulation boost, eases the internal congestion, brings a "youth awakening" to the prostate gland, and helps promote youthful hormones. Following this bath, rub yourself dry and warm up with a coarse Turkish towel.

3. *Contrast Sitz Bath.* This calls for two tubs—or else, you may work quickly to change from hot to cold. Fill the tub only midway with hot water and sit with your knees drawn up, for 10 to 15 minutes. Then quickly change to comfortably cold water for just *one minute.* Then change back to the comfortably hot water for 10 to 15 minutes. Again, change quickly to the comfortably cold water for just one minute. Try to make up to five such contrast changes. Always finish with the cold water. *Benefit:* The contrast of hot-cold water has a "glandular massage" effect, alerting the sluggish circulation and helping the rhythmic gland clocks to issue forth a supply of healing hormones. When the prostate gland is thus alerted by the contrast of hot-cold water, it is able to function more healthfully, promoting youth in this most vital region of the male body.

The simple Sitz Bath has brought new life to sleepy prostate glands for tens of thousands of men. For many of them, the all-natural Sitz Bath has replaced artificial stimulants or chemical pills. This tends to prove that the health of the body is in the health of the glands. When the prostate and other glands were alerted by water therapy, the entire body enjoyed a feeling of "hormonized" youth and vigor. These programs are finding their way into our modern healing institutions throughout the world.

Six Benefits of the "Nature Water" Shower

A most rejuvenating and health-restoring water program is that of the "Nature Water" Shower which calls for the use of the old-fashioned but exhilarating cold water soaking. By using comfortably cold water in a nature-created temperature, it has this set of glandular benefits:

1. A cold water shower increases glandular circulation, strengthens muscular tone, and alerts the hormones to soothe the nervous system.
2. The adrenal glands react to external stimuli, such as nature-temperature cold water. A cold water shower will alert this gland to issue forth natural healing hormones and help alert the connecting network of endocrines to work in rhythmic hormone harmony.
3. Digestive glands wake up to the stimuli of cold water, sending forth metabolic hormones to boost the powers of assimilation and digestion.
4. The adrenal-pituitary glands become awakened by cold water, improving and strengthening the central nervous system, sending "young" hormones to the brain, bearing youth-building oxygen to other vital organs, creating a "forever young" feeling.
5. Cold water sends young hormones to the respiratory region, to nourish the delicate membranes, cells, and tissues, to help build resistance to winter ailments and nasal-throat allergies.
6. The "Nature Water" Shower is comfortably cold, helping to adjust the body temperature to that of nature. This regulating of the body's thermostat further helps adjust the biological gland clocks. The hormones nourish and stimulate the body's organs and promote a youthful feeling.

The "Nature Water" Shower is known as a "youth elixir" because of its hormone-alerting function. It's easy—and free!

How Bridget K. Became Young Through the "Nature Water"

Shower. In a reported case, Bridget K. looked pale, was susceptible to allergies, had weakened digestive powers, was nervous, edgy, and had embarrassing constipation. She was put on a natural health program and given wholesome hormone foods. Bridget K. enjoyed natural sweets and herbal spices on a no-salt, no-sugar program. She responded with a bloom in her cheeks, but her healing was incomplete until she followed a twice-daily "Nature Water" Shower. She would stand beneath a cold shower for just 10 minutes. The cold water on her face alerted sluggish hormones to awaken, to help smooth out wrinkles, causing an electronic-like revitalization. Furthermore, *the cold water helped the hormones transport more oxygen to her blood cells, improving her basic health and appearance.*

Bridget K. followed this natural program, with the twice-daily "Nature Water" Shower, for over two weeks. She emerged with resistance against allergies, a better digestive power, a happy temperament, and freedom from constipation. She felt young. She looked young. Indeed, the "Nature Water" Shower program had given her a generous supply of young hormones. Now she had much to live for again.

How to Take a Sea-Water Bath in Your Own Tub

The seas are rich in minerals that are absorbed through the skin and help nourish the glands. Many people who spent a few days at the seashore have experienced an invigorating benefit—a youthful vitality and a sparkle of youthfulness in the eyes. Furthermore, the mineral-rich seaside air also sends a stream of "mineral vapors" through the nostrils; this mineral-rich oxygen is absorbed by the hormones, thereby enriching their youth-making powers. If you can go to the seashore, do so as regularly as possible. As a substitute, at home, fill your tub with water and dissolve one cup of Epsom salt, together with one cup of common salt. Then immerse yourself in this comfortably tepid tub. The minerals from the salts will help approximate the benefit from the open seas. It is as close to the real thing as possible. The benefit here is that these minerals will enter through the pores and be taken up by the glands, which then metabolize them into usable nutritives for the hormones. Thus, the hormones have a youthfully enriched power that will help boost overall body-mind health.

The Herbal Bath for Glandular Adjustment

Into pleasantly warm water, place a handful of any available herbs such as some fragrant pine, eucalyptus, mint, rosemary, sage, alfalfa, or fenugreek. Let the herbs soak for about 10 minutes in a tub of comfortably warm water. Then soak yourself in this fragrant water up to 30 minutes.

Those who have taken this Herbal Bath should emerge with a satisfied feeling of soothing relaxation. Tense and nervous limbs should be relaxed. There should now be a restoration of the internal equilibrium that makes life a joyful experience.

Secret: The substances in the herbs help soothe the endocrine glands, especially the inter-related adrenal-pituitary. When these herbs soothe the glands, there is a rhythmic glandular adjustment of hormones that creates a soothing balance of emotional health. The Herbal Bath has been called nature's own "brain tonic." The action on the glands help soothe and relax the neuro-muscular and brain chain to promote healing hormones.

The Bavarian Oil Bath for "Glandular Rebirth"

Hattie E. was in her early 50's, but she was mistaken for being in her 70's. In a reported case, she developed arthritic-like stiffness and would wear heavy garments, even in warm weather, because of "chills." She walked with a stooped gait. Her memory was faulty. At times, she would forget what she wanted to say, right in the middle of a sentence. Hattie E. went to such a health "water" resort, and was put on a unique glandular rebirth program as follows:

1. *Raw Juice Fast.* One day a week, Hattie E. went on a raw juice fast. She would drink fresh, raw juices for breakfast; mid-day, a vegetable juice cocktail. For lunch, a combination of different raw vegetable juices. Mid-afternoon, a fresh fruit juice pickup. For dinner, a raw vegetable juice cocktail with a sprinkle of lemon juice. The benefit here is that this helped cleanse the system and wash the glands of accumulated debris.

2. *Oil Bath Daily.* Hattie E. took a Bavarian Oil Bath every single day. Into a tub of comfortably warm water was poured one cup of corn oil (or olive oil), one tablespoon of any liquid detergent shampoo, and one teaspoon of oil of rose geranium or any desired

perfume. When mixed together, the warm water helped the oil break down into millions of tiny oil globules. The nutrients in the oil were helped to enter into the pores cleansed by the shampoo (some 7 million of them dot the skin surface) and were sent streaming to the tired glands. Hattie E.'s entire endocrine system was thus treated to the Bavarian Oil Bath, alerting sluggish glands so they sent forth youth-building hormones.

3. *Wholesome Foods.* Hattie's corrective hormone food program called for wholesome foods—no fragments, such as processed, chemicalized, adulterated foods. Everything had to be as wholesome and natural as possible. The purpose was to help readjust the tired glands, to help establish a bio-rhythmic hormonal flow.

4. *Nightly Sleep.* Hattie E. was told to obtain a full night of rest, without fail. The glands needed sleep just as the other body organs did. This helped rest the glands and enabled them to awaken feeling refreshed and rejuvenated, able to greet the new day with healthful hormone-making values.

Improvement Progress: It took several weeks before Hattie E. experienced improvement. Her posture was improved, her memory was more alert, her "chills" subsided, and she felt warm and pleasantly stimulated. Her arthritic-like limbs felt less painful. She was well on the way to recovery.

How to Relax Your Glands to Promote Healthful Sleep

Many visitors to the water cure health spas, and those who frequent the modern health resorts, complain of nervous unrest, edgy nerves, irritation at little noises, chronic fatigue, as well as health-depleting insomnia. The key to gland-healing sleep is to relax the body from *within* as well as from *without*. Spa practitioners have noted that the "gland relaxing" bath is able to promote overall relaxation and an invitation to healthful sleep, without medicines.

The Spa Bath for Gland-Inducing Sleep. Fill a tub with water, about 100-102°F, just several degrees above the body's own temperature. NOTE: The temperature should be neither too hot nor too cold. Fill the tub so you can lie within, completely submerged, right up to your chin. Place a rolled-up towel or a plastic-covered cushion behind your head. The nape of your neck should be comfortably supported by the towel to promote soothing relaxation. Rest in this

Spa Bath for 30 minutes. *Unique Benefits:* The warm water relaxes the adrenal-pituitary glands to help draw tension and congestion. away from the inner organs. The Spa Bath helps these glands send soothing hormones to relax the blood vessels, stabilize the circulation, and help send a flush of nourishing red blood to the entire body. In the simple Spa Bath, the soothing hormones *force* the body to relax.

Just 10 to 15 minutes will begin to relax the blood pressure, soothe the nerve endings with balm-like hormones that form a stress shield over the raw edges, and help promote relaxed and deep breathing.

Step out of the Spa Bath with relaxed glands, pat (don't rub) yourself gently dry, and then ease into bed for deep and tranquil sleep.

Father Kneipp and his successor-practitioners have reported much success in easing jangled nerves by relaxing the biological gland clocks through healthful foods and tranquilizing water baths.

The Sulphur Bath for Arthritis Relief

Father Kneipp recommended the use of sulphur baths. The benefit here is that this mineral is able to soothe the glands, enter into the adrenal hormones, and promote a cortisone-like relief for twisted or painful joints and limbs. Many who came to his water cure spa, experienced remarkable arthritis relief on the natural food programs *and* the daily Sulphur Bath. In our modern times, the Sulphur Bath may be enjoyed right in your own home.

How to Make Your Own Sulphur Bath: To a tub filled with 25 gallons of water (average tub capacity), add just two ounces of *potassium sulphide.* This sulphur powder is available at most herbal and other pharmacies. Dissolve this mineral, then immerse yourself into the comfortably warm water and remain up to 30 minutes. *Arthritis-Easing Benefit:* Sulphur and other minerals seep through the skin pores and enter into the fluid-filled inter-cellular spaces of the body's glands. Here, the minerals join with gland-making hormones and add more value to these internal rivers. When the adrenal-pituitary glands secrete their cortisone-like hormones, these liquids are enriched with sulphur and other minerals which work to help soothe the painful joints and limbs. Such a Sulphur Bath was mandatory for all arthritic patients going to the health spa. It is reported that many emerged from such programs with the remark that the bath was like a "fountain of youth" in modern times. The enriched hormones had worked their rejuvenating benefits upon the entire body and limbs, helping to create better flexibility and ease of movement.

The Sulphur Bath, like others used at the health spa, have a favorable action on the hormone circulation and send soothing hormones into the tiny arteries, veins, and capillaries throughout the body, from head to toe, bringing new life and health to every body cell.

The great healing power of water may be in the "peripheral hormonal circulation" throughout the entire body. When the water cure baths are followed together with natural health programs, the body's gland clocks have a chance to become precision-timed, to be able to send forth a rhythmic river of youth-building hormones. Nature has put great healing power into water. This all-natural, gland-boosting tonic may well be the "hormone supplement" of the future.

Highlights

1. Father Kneipp's "living water" programs helped improve glandular health and promoted the vigor of natural hormones.

2. The time-tested Sitz Bath offers soothing comfort to the male prostate gland.

3. A simple "Nature Water" Shower offers six gland-boosting benefits.

4. How to take a Sea-Water Bath in your own tub at home.

5. How the Herbal Bath helps create glandular adjustment.

6. Hattie E. became young again with a Bavarian Oil Bath and natural health program.

7. The Sulphur Bath reportedly helps promote natural cortisone through glandular awakening, thereby easing arthritic distress naturally.

16

Six Special Hormone Food Programs to Strengthen the Gland-Hormone Network for Youthful Health

Youthful health is directed by a well-nourished glandular system. In particular, the degree of enjoying a "feel young for life" vitality is influenced by the health of the hormones produced by the endocrine glands. These hormones possess the secret of extended youth. These same hormones blend in with more glandular secretions to promote an internal *bio-electronic principle,* which provides youthful stimulus to your body and alertness to your mind.

The *bio-electronic principle* becomes activated by proper food programs, in conjunction with natural health living, to help improve the quality and quantity of hormones that enter into most vital life processes and build resistance to premature and unnecessary aging. These same food programs help promote a healthy functioning of your endocrine glands, alert this *bio-electronic principle* right within your own body, and keep your hormones in good working rhythm. To energize the hormone-improving abilities of the endocrine glands, nature has placed "nourishment" in the form of hormone foods to help "pull the switch" of the *bio-electronic principle* of the body. In particular, six special hormone food programs are known for establishing an internal equilibrium that promotes nourishment of the endocrine glandular system and helps this network send forth a healthful supply of youth-producing hormones. *Special Benefit:* The *bio-electronic principle* is as vigorous and effective as the foods you eat. By following the natural health programs in this book, as well as the six special hormone food programs in this chapter, you will be feeding your glands, alerting the *bio-electronic principle* that sends forth a rich and well-nourished supply of youth-building hormones. The following six food programs are especially beneficial in adjusting this principle to set off a rhythmic balance of youth-building hormones.

Gland-Feeding Program #1—*Brewer's Yeast*

Locked within a tiny yeast cell are the richest known sources of the B-complex vitamins; they enter into the feeding of the glandular cells and tissues and are found in the composition of the hormones themselves. The yeast cell has been prepared in a wholesome and natural food known as Brewer's Yeast. It has 17 different vitamins, including all those of the B-complex family, some 16 amino acids, about 14 minerals, and a goodly assortment of digestive enzymes. This wonder food has long been hailed as a gland food because it has been able to reportedly give more energy to housewives, promote more vigor in salesmen, teachers, and active people in all walks of life, and increase stamina and morale. Its bio-electronic principle in boosting a healthful supply of hormones is so effective, that Brewer's Yeast has reportedly been said to help people retain the characteristics of youth at all ages!

How Brewer's Yeast Promotes Production of Youth-Building Hormones. The substances in Brewer's Yeast are taken up by the endocrine glands and sent streaming into the hormone-carrying bloodstream to help enrich the intra-cellular tissues and cells of the body's organs and the skin itself. Here, the hormones help enrich the delicate tissues, send nourishment to the fragile cells, pep up action of the sluggish blood sugar, promote internal healing, and restore tired blood corpuscles.

The miniscule, 1/4,000th-of-an-inch-in-diameter Brewer's Yeast cell contains nearly all of the substances that are found right in the body's own hormones! Microscopic, the yeast cell has the powers of "budding" or rejuvenation at an astonishingly speedy rate. It is this self-rejuvenation power that is so valuable to the hormones, which then take up this miracle youth-building principle and help provide it to the body itself. The secret of the hormone "youthification" benefit of Brewer's Yeast is in its own regenerative powers that are then provided to the system itself. Brewer's Yeast is truly one of nature's most important "living" gland foods.

How a Schoolteacher Recharges Her Glands in Mid-Afternoon. Early afternoon is a fatigue spot for Betty K., a hard-working schoolteacher. She looked for a quick-and-easy hormone food "pick-up" that would help recharge her glands so that she could continue teaching throughout the afternoon and still have healthful energy at the end of the day. She followed the basic natural health programs, and then boosted her hormone-energizing supply by preparing a tasty and effective *Mid-Afternoon Hormone Food Recharger.* Here is how Betty K. prepares it:

In one glass of fruit or vegetable juice, or even in one glass of milk, mix together four heaping tablespoons of Brewer's Yeast powder. Stir vigorously. Drink slowly.

Benefits: The vitamins and minerals join with the amino acids to help alert the bio-electronic principle in the glands, which then become healthfully awakened to send forth a more enriched supply of energy-building hormones. These hormones, enriched with the "budding" or self-reproducing powers of the yeast cells, work to bathe and wash the body's organs and help promote a feeling of energy and vitality. Just one such glass of *Mid-Afternoon Hormone Food Recharger*, in combination with a natural health program, has made Betty K. a "new woman," and "a young one at that," in the latter part of the day, when other schoolteachers feel tired and look wan. The enriched hormones have given her a new and youthful lease on life.

How to Feed Brewer's Yeast to Your Glands. Available in tablets or powder, you may take this all-natural gland food regularly with fresh fruit or vegetable juice or a glass of milk. You may use four heaping teaspoons of yeast daily as a mixture with seed oil for your raw vegetable salad dressing. You may stir the powder in soups, stews, and sauces. TIP: Sprinkle a teaspoon of Brewer's Yeast powder in one cup of fresh yogurt for a hormone-enrichment benefit that will make you love life with youthful anticipation. You may also obtain Brewer's Yeast in handy tablet form to be taken daily with fresh juices.

This tiny yeast cell reportedly has the wholesome ability to help alert the bio-electronic principles that promote glandular rejuvenation and healthy hormones. Many regard it as a "wonder" food for the glands.

Gland-Feeding Program #2—*Miracle Magnesium*

A lesser-known but highly effective mineral that helps feed the glands with more benefits than the other nutrients is that of *magnesium*, often called "the hormone mineral of life" because it helps feed the glands in such a remarkable way.

How Magnesium Helps Keep the Brain Feeling Young. The hormones take this metabolized mineral and use it to help the motor nerves (those that carry messages by electric impulse from the brain to the muscles) send out their minute electric charges. Magnesium-nourished hormones can spell the difference between sluggish or so-called senile mentality or quick, smooth, and well-coordinated youthful brain power. Many scientists have labelled this "miracle mineral" as a "hormone memory food" because the hormones use it to help improve the memory functions of the mind and boost a youthful thinking capacity.

How Magnesium-Nourished Hormones Rejuvenate Brain Cells. The hormones need magnesium to help nourish tiny substances within the brain cells. Known as *mitochondria*, these substances require energy from the magnesium in the hormones that wash into the brain cells.

Such youthful "thinking energies" come from magnesium-nourished hormones which work to activate enzymes to help oxidate glucose and produce "thought" and "intelligence." The magnesium is used by the hormones to work with enzymes to produce this youthful brain response. The magnesium empowers the hormones to mediate the movement of muscles, the process of breathing, the storage of energy, the digestion of food, the building of tissues, the course of reproduction, the transmission of nerve impulses, and the youthful workings of the brain. The magnesium helps the hormones rejuvenate the thought processes themselves!

This miracle mineral healthfully stimulates the hormones to help boost the youth-building abilities of the neuron-brain system.

How Magnesium Created Hormone-Rejuvenated Nerves. In one reported case, a group of patients with malnourished endocrines, displayed symptoms of nervous unrest, mental irrationalism, and prematurely aging emotions. When examined, these patients were found to have sluggish glands, and, in particular, a magnesium deficiency in the hormones.

Unique Recovery Program. The patients were given magnesium food supplements. In about three months, when the hormone deficient patients followed natural health principles and magnesium supplementation, they now became youthful, active, cooperative, congenial people. Their emotions were stable and youthful. The miracle mineral, magnesium, had alerted their glands and nourished their hormones to promote rejuvenated nerves.

Special Note: In a condition of magnesium deficiency, the glands are forced to draw on tissue reserves and deplete stored up minerals. The glands must turn "cannibal" and devour their own magnesium source. Hence, magnesium must always be available in an abundant supply, so that the glands need not drain out their valuable reserves and upset their delicate time-precision availability to the hormones.

Natural Gland-Feeding Sources of Magnesium: Just one-half of an average cup of these foods daily offers the glands a high supply of this miracle mineral:

Almonds	.252 milligrams
Barley, whole	.171
Beans, dried lima	.181
Beet greens	.113
Brazil nuts	.225
Cashew nuts	.267
Corn	.121
Endive	.380
Honey	.386
Kohlrabi	.370
Rice, brown	.119
Wheat germ	.511

SUGGESTION: Sunflower seeds have some 350 milligrams of magnesium (together with a treasure of hormone-enriching vitamins, minerals, enzymes, and proteins) in just one-half cupful. You would do well to munch about one-half cup of sunflower seeds daily.

How Magnesium Feeds the Pituitary Gland. This miracle mineral is food for the pituitary gland. (The pea-sized gland at the base of the brain.) Magnesium helps energize the pituitary to take instructions from the hypothalamus, then transmit these impulses through the body. The hormones carry magnesium to help influence the physiological-emotional processes and also enter into the balanced production of other body hormones.

The pituitary must have its supply of magnesium; a deficiency of this natural food means that the pituitary weakens in its control over other organisms. There may be internal upheaval. Often, the endocrines become hyper-excited and this creates tensions and nervous, erratic behavior symptoms. But with magnesium, the pituitary can help maintain youthful emotional tranquility.

Unique Youth Benefit: Magnesium is used by the hormones to feed energy to the motor nerves, feed the central nervous system, stabilize the spinal cord, regulate the nervous system, and enter into the hormone-balancing effects of the blood levels.

How to Feed Magnesium to Your Glands: The natural hormone foods listed above should be part of the daily hormone food program. Magnesium is also available in supplemental form, and in all-purpose mineral tablets sold at most pharmacies and health food shops. *Suggestion:* Eat dark green, leafy vegetables, all soybean products, nuts, cashews, almonds, Brazil nuts, pumpkin seeds, and whole grains. TIP: Eat these foods *raw* and *non-processed* since cooking leads to a loss of much magnesium.

Gland-Feeding Program #3—*Gelatine*

A popular hormone food is that of gelatine, which is made from the dried bones of cattle, prepared in a form that may be stirred into a glass of fruit or vegetable juice and taken as a "hormone cocktail," or it may be used as a gelatine dessert.

Special Hormone-Boosting Benefits of Gelatine. The glands take up the amino acids from the metabolized gelatine protein, use them to nourish the bloodstream, enrich the tissues, rejuvenate the organs, smooth the skin, nourish the hair, and feed the fibres of the nails. Hormones take these amino acids to feed the nerves and brain and help promote a healthful feeling of overall improvement in body and mind.

Unique Youth-Restorative Benefits of Hormone-Enriched Protein. The hormone-enriched protein enters into the bloodstream to help make healthy tissue over that which has been broken down or otherwise injured. The protein from gelatine is used by the hormones to help strengthen the cells of the muscles and boost a feeling of energy and vitality.

The hormones, themselves, are made up of the very same amino acids found in gelatine. The hormones need this all-natural wholesome food to help create the bio-electronic forces of youthful health.

How Protein Hormones Resist Illness. The protein hormones work to create natural gamma globulin (a blood protein that forms antibodies which neutralize bacteria, viruses, and other micro-organisms). Protein hormones make gamma globulin, to help promote immunity by engulfing and destroying disease microbes.

These protein-nourished hormones help create antibodies in the bloodstream to help neutralize unhealthy virus invasions, build youthful resistance, and stimulate recovery from the ravages of debilitation.

Daily Protein, a Hormone "Must." A constant turnover makes adequate daily protein a hormone "must." The turnover is faster within the cells of a tissue (intra-cellular) than in the substance between the cells (inter-cellular), and hormones must have a healthful supply of the protein to maintain this delicate and life- health-building balance.

How to Feed Gelatine Protein to Your Glands: To obtain an adequate supply of daily protein, remember to eat foods such as meat, fish, eggs, cheese, peas, beans, nuts, and whole grains. But, in particular, *gelatine* is a highly beneficial "gland food" because it is a prime source of nearly all of the essential amino acids or metabolized protein needed to feed your endocrine glands with youthful nourishment.

"GIFT OF LIFE" GLAND FOOD. Into one glass of freshly prepared vegetable juice, stir four heaping tablespoons of *unflavored* gelatine. Stir vigorously. *Optional:* A squeeze of lemon juice for a piquant taste. Drink just one glass daily to instill a "gift of life" feeling in the body's endocrine glands. This "Gift of Life" Gland Food is a prime source of those very amino acids needed by the hormones to help create a feeling of youthful health and overall fitness.

Gland-Feeding Program #4—*Raw Juices*

Natural, raw, fresh fruit and vegetable juices are rich sources of nutrients as well as enzymes that are needed by the glands to help promote a feeling of youthful health. These same nutrients, and enzymes, are found within the hormones, themselves. A deficiency may lead to weakened hormones which will have less ability to keep the body and mind in a healthful condition. Just as enzymes are found in all living substances, so do they promote "life" to the hormones, when introduced in the form of natural, raw, and non-processed juices.

Five Gland-Feeding Benefits of Raw Juices. The five most outstanding benefits of raw juices are these:

1. Enzymes in raw juices work through the hormones to help enrich the bloodstream and build a youthful internal "river of life."

Since hormones gush directly into the bloodstream, it is healthful to have a good supply of enzymes which are needed by the bloodstream for promoting regeneration in the body from head to toe.

2. The blood utilizes the enzyme-enriched hormones to absorb oxygen in the lungs and distribute this "breath of life" to every organ, every body part. The blood then uses the enzyme-enriched hormones to carry a cargo of age-causing carbon dioxide wastes, which go to the lungs for disposal.

3. Enzyme-enriched hormones carry other age-causing waste products from the body tissues to the kidneys, which filter out the wastes into the urine.

4. On their way through the body, the enzymes in the hormones help gather up nutrients and water from the digested food in the in estines and bring these nutrients to the tissues and cells. This is the vital regeneration process that is created when the hormones have healthful enzymes.

5. Enzymes in the bloodstream work to transport the body's other hormones from their glands to wherever they are needed to help improve health and youth.

Today, researchers are convinced that a vast majority of age-causing conditions of ill health may be traced to a deficiency of enzymes in the hormones.

How to Feed Enzymes to Your Glands: Each day, drink fresh, raw fruit and vegetable juices. Here are several enzyme-rich juices that help nourish your glands and your body-mind combination:

Wonder-Worker Hormone Punch. Mix equal portions of grape juice, berry juice, and apple juice. Squeeze two tablespoons of lemon juice into the glass. Stir vigorously. Drink as a "juice break" instead of coffee in mid-morning. *The Wonder-Worker Hormone Punch* has a rich supply of vitamins and minerals that work with the enzyme-plus content to boost the health of the glands and enrich the hormones that promote youthful vitality.

Hormone Food Delight. Mix one pint of tomato juice, one glass of carrot juice, and one-half glass of berry juice. Stir vigorously. Season with a sprinkle of vegetized salt or sea salt (kelp). Drink one glass in the morning, the balance in portions throughout the day. The *Hormone Food Delight* has a well-balanced supply of nutrients that help pep up sluggish glands and promote a healthy feeling of body and mind.

"E" Bomb for Hormone Vitality. One glass of skim milk, two tablespoons of dark organic honey, two teaspoons of Brewer's Yeast

powder, and two teaspoons of dark molasses. Stir vigorously or put under blender. The *"E" Bomb for Hormone Vi ality* is a potent blending of valuable enzymes and inter-related nutrients that offer peedy assimilation by the glands to help promote hormone vitality. *TIP:* Try it for a lunch—all by itself. It reportedly help tir up sleepy glands to boost the body-mind functions for most of the afternoon—nature's own gland tonic!

Natural, raw fruit and vegetable juices should form the foundation for glandular regeneration. Drink these juices regulary. Your glands will be glad you did!

Gland-Feeding Program #5—*Hormone Oils*

Natural seed oils carry with them the precious unsaturated fatty acids and the recognized Vitamin E that is necessary food or the glands. In particular, seed and vegetable oils are needed by the hormones to help promote energy, put a sparkle in the eyes, spare the heart's use of oxygen, and send a stream of fresh hormones to the brain in order to promote youthful thinking processes. In natural seed and vegetable oils, nature has given us a supply of "hormone foods" that help boost life, health, and youthful alertness.

How Oils Help Ease Symptoms of Premature Aging. The body's glands extract substances from oils which are sent into the hormones. These enriched hormones pour into the bloodstream, which uses these substances to enter into the blood vessels (capillaries) of the muscles and heart tissue, the arteries, and the various bio-chemical processes of the entire body.

The oils are used to conserve body oxygen and become an *electron-carrier* of health to the body's organs. The hormones use these electron-carriers to help influence the glycogen metabolism, the healthful digestive process, and the overall assimilation of food to help produce health for the body and mind. Small wonder that seed and vegetable oils are known as "hormone oils" because they are used to promote internal regeneration and "lubrication" of vital functions.

Hormones prefer these liquid oils, which are easier to process and are not deposited as fat unless you are overeating.

How to Feed Oil to Your Glands. Use as a salad dressing. *TIP:* Follow the time-tested European secret of blending two-thirds liquid oil to one-third apple cider vinegar. This is a tasty and delicious way to feed oil to your glands.

Golden Oil Health Brew: Into one glass of raw vegetable juice, stir four tablespoons of wheat germ oil. A squeeze of lemon juice helps create a pleasantly tart flavor. Stir vigorously. Sip slowly. *Benefit:* The minerals combine with the Vitamin E to help create a healthful balance that is readily taken up by the glands, and offered to the hormones in a form that is comfortably utilized.

Breakfast Booster: Have a large raw vegetable salad for breakfast. Sprinkle four tablespoons of cold-pressed wheat germ oil on top of the vegetables. Sprinkle wheat germ flakes for added Vitamin E benefits. The availability of unsaturated fatty acids and Vitamin E in the early morning is healthful for the still-sleepy glands, and may well help promote "energetic hormones" to see you through the morning with youthful vigor.

Hormones need oils as a means of lubrication and resilient flexibility. Help boost the *bio-electronic principles* of the endocrine glandular network with these golden oils of nature.

Gland-Feeding Program #6—*Rice*

Your glands need carbohydrates for energy. The secret here is to feed them natural and wholesome carbohydrates from natural and wholesome foods. One historic food is that of *rice.* The Orientals have long known that natural brown rice is nature's almost "perfect" food because it is capable of offering a treasure of hormone nourishment for life and health. Although rice is a prime source of many substances, it is not to be eaten as a sole item. That is, it is *part* of the gland-feeding program but should not be eaten to the exclusion of other foods. Nature has created a bountiful supply of many foods that work in harmony to help nourish the glands and promote youthful hormones. Eat all foods in healthful balance for a healthful glandular network. Rice is one of the various foods needed by the glands for helping to promote carbohydrate-energized hormones.

What Rice Will Do to Nourish the Glands. Natural brown rice will nourish the glands by helping to bring rice protein (contains eight out of 11 essential amino acids) to the hormones. Rice will also send the B-complex vitamins into the hormones to provide youthful energy and nourish the skin and blood vessels.

Rice sends minerals to the hormones to be used to heal wounds, create a healthy heartbeat, and stabilize blood pressure.

NOTE: Natural brown rice sends phosphorus and potassium into the hormones, which are needed to metabolize other nutrients and maintain internal water balance.

Hormones Use Rice Nourishment to Regenerate Digestion. The glands offer a unique rice substance to the hormones—*amylopectin.* This natural rice substance, amylopectin, is used by the hormones to promote a youthful and speedy digestion. For those who are troubled with "middle-aged digestion," this rice substance is needed by the hormones to help improve-regenerate the so-called faulty digestion.

Hormones welcome substances in rice because they are soothing and healing and virtually salt-free to help maintain a natural balance.

Rice has a natural and unique type of carbohydrate that is easily handled by the digestive system and is a form of "quick energy" for the glands. The Orientals knew that brown rice was healthful and often regarded it as a "youth food"; hence, their record of longevity which is unsurpassed even in our modern countries. Rice may well be the "hormone food" that offers most youthful nourishment to the glandular network.

How to Feed Rice Nourishment to Your Glands: Select natural brown rice. This is the whole, unpolished grain of rice, with only the outer hull and a small amount of bran removed. It has a delightful, nut-like flavor and a slightly chewy texture. Eat rice at least three times a week, as a side dish with a meal, or as a between-meal snack. And—a bowl of steaming rice with a dollop of honey and a glass of fresh fruit juice is a wonderful breakfast!

Oven-Baked Rice: Heat oven to 350°F. Combine one cup of uncooked brown rice and two cups of water into a three-quart baking dish. Cover. Bake 25-30 minutes, or until rice is tender.

Feathered Rice Method. Heat oven to 375°F. Spread one cup of rice in a shallow baking pan. Bake, stirring occasionally, until rice grains are golden brown. Remove pan from oven. Now turn oven heat to 400°F. Put toasted rice into one-and-a-half quart casserole dish with a tight-fitting cover. Stir in two-and-a-half cups of boiling water. Cover. Bake 20 minutes.

Double Boiler Rice. When rice is cooked in milk, it is most frequently cooked over boiling water; that is, in the top of a double boiler. Place one cup of natural brown rice in the top of a double boiler with three-and-a-half cups of milk. Heat to boiling, then place over boiling water, and cook, covered, for 40 minutes, or until milk is absorbed.

As an important natural carbohydrate food, rice may well be the "energy booster" needed by the glands to help promote a feeling of youthful health. Take a tip from the long-living, "young" Orientals and feed rice to your glands!

Essential Chapter Points

1. Alert the youth-building, bio-electronic principles of the endocrines by natural living and emphasis upon six special food programs that feed your glands with energy and vigor.

2. Brewer's Yeast feeds vitamins to the hormones.

3. Magnesium is a "miracle mineral" that creates mental-physical balance in a unique glandular rhythm.

4. Simple gelatine offers "instant" protein to the glands.

5. Natural, raw fruit and vegetable juices send living enzymes to the body's endocrine glands and hormones to promote youthful vitality.

6. Hormone oils are found in natural seed and plant juices.

7. The Orientals use natural brown rice as an "energy food" for the glands and enjoy prolonged youth through "forever young" hormones.

17

Hormone Herbs: Nature's Secrets of Youthful Gland Action

The great remedial and youthful hormone proper-
ties of herbs have been recognized and appreciated by all civilizations
since time immemorial. The ancients looked to the gardens and fields
for their natural organic medicines from the plant kingdom. Here
were hundreds of herbs that could be brewed in tasty hot or cold
beverages, to be sipped with delicious enjoyment along with hormone-feeding benefits. In these herbs, nature has placed a treasure of
folklore healing with glandular nourishment, that has made them a
veritable "garden of youth."

Sealed within the flowers, roots, bark, and leaves of nature's
"grass medicines" are hormone-like substances that help adjust the
body's biological gland clocks, helping them issue forth their secretions of healthfulness. These substances may well be nature's own
"hormone supplements." Many long-recognized herbs contain those
very substances of which hormones are made! Small wonder that
nature's grasses have long been used as "hormone herbs."

The Indian Herb That Boosts the Health of the Blood-Building Gland

Slippery elm was the food and blood-building natural medicine of
the American Indians and the pioneers. Native to the United States,
it was most abundant west of the Allegheny Mountain range. The
Indians regarded it as a "blood building" herb and were known to

drink it in the form of an infusion of tea, almost regularly, with amazing benefits.

Although the Indians had no knowledge of the blood-building function of the adrenal glands, they noticed that a tea made of slippery elm was pleasantly sweet and helped produce a warm feeling as well as a more youthfully healthy color in the infirm.

Slippery elm was much in use amongst the American Indians and has maintained its value today for those who seek a natural herbal way to help boost the action of "tired" glands."

How an Herb-Activated Adrenal Gland Put Roses in a Secretary's Cheeks. A sallow complexion and a generally "cold hands and cold feet" feeling made Janet A. look and feel much older than she was. This secretary was told that she had a "sluggish adrenal problem" but was unable to take inorganic (chemicalized) medicines because of side effects and sensations of vertigo (dizziness).

All Janet A. could do was soak her hands and feet in hot water, almost nightly, with temporary relief. Next morning, she would still have that cold sensation in her fingers and toes. Her sallow, somewhat blotchy skin was a further sign of poor health.

Janet A. might have endured her prematurely aging appearance, had she not come across some paragraphs of Indian herbalism in a book she was reading about the Old West. She learned that the American Indians and early pioneers would use nature's grasses to help boost their health and put color into pale bodies.

Unique Gland Benefit. Janet A. read of slippery elm as one herb that reportedly boosted the health of the adrenal glands. When slippery elm was made in an infusion of tea, it released several hormone-like substances directly to the adrenal glands, gave a "boost" to the cortex (outer layer), and helped improve the natural flow of *cortin,* the hormone that helps build rich, healthy blood. Janet A. decided to try this special Indian herb.

Blood-Building Hormone Tea. To make slippery elm tea at home Janet A. obtained a powdered form from a local herbal pharmacy. She dissolved just one-half teaspoon of powdered slippery elm bark in one cup of boiled water. She added a tablespoon of milk and one teaspoon of natural honey for sweetening. Janet A. drank this special all-natural Blood-Building Hormone Tea, at least three times daily.

Benefit: Ingredients in the herb helped assist the activity of the adrenal glands. Specifically, the herbal ingredients gently helped to revive the cortex of the adrenals, thus boosting the output of the cortin hormone; this helped send a stream of blood-building substances that warmed the hands and feet and promoted a feeling of youth throughout the body.

Looks and Feels Younger. The Blood-Building Hormone Tea, along with an emphasis upon natural foods and natural health programs, helped Janet's adrenal glands promote a youthful warmth. Now she looked and felt younger. She also had the bloom of roses in her cheeks. She felt like the picture of flowering youth, thanks to the American Indian herbal remedy. This secretary still follows the natural health programs that emphasize herbal teas, and she enjoys the healthy benefits of a properly adjusted hormonal network.

The Mediterranean Herb That Relaxes "Stiff Fingers"

The simple, yet highly effective parsley herb is a native of Sardinia and other parts of Southern Europe, where it has long been hailed as a "miracle healer" because of its ability to relax "stiff fingers" or "gnarled joints" that are likened to arthritic-rheumatic symptoms.

Parsley root has been found to contain all-natural ingredients that help produce an anodyne (pain-relieving) benefit to relax stiff fingers and joints and promote more youthful flexibility of the limbs. This herb is a rich source of vitamins as well as four vital minerals (calcium, copper, iron, and manganese) that work in a unique *harmony* to help create a hormone-like benefit to stiff "pockets" in the system. In this nature-created, balanced *harmony*, parsley root is able to promote relaxation and general easing of "tightness."

The Secret of Parsley Action: Reportedly parsley offers a welcome supply of speedily assimilated Vitamin A that is taken up by the glands to help regulate a smooth hormonal rhythm throughout the body. This *meatless source* of Vitamin A may well be nature's major secret of youthful health. It helps relax the tightness of internal congestion. Parsley is a Greek word meaning "stone breaker" which indicates that the ancients were well aware of this hormone herb for its soothing benefits.

How Parsley Root Tea Gave New Life to a Dressmaker's Stiff Fingers. Bertha K. earned her living as a dressmaker. When her fingers became stiff and unmanageable, she grew frightened. The gnarled sensation made it increasingly difficult for her to thread a needle or operate her sewing machine. Faced with the problem of inflexible fingers and wrists, she tried inorganic medication. This helped ease her symptoms, but her joints still felt stiff and gnarled.

It was through conversation with a European customer that she heard of legendary and time-tested hormone herbs. She heard of the parsley root herb and how so many folks would use this "organic medicine" to help promote youthful flexibility in their limbs.

Bertha K. scoffed at such "old wives' tales." But her customer took pity on her and brought the slow-working dressmaker a month's supply of this herb. She insisted that Bertha K. drink this tea daily.

At first, Bertha K. felt some relief. It took several weeks before she was able to experience a gradual and gentle "unstiffening" of her fingers and thumbs. Her wrists still had a thickening sensation, but she was encouraged in that her stiffness began to relax. In a few months, when following a natural health program, elimination of white sugar, white flour, salt, and processed foods, along with nightly rest and parsley root tea, Bertha K. could thread a needle as easily and expertly as in her younger days. She had learned to trust in nature's herbal hormones as her best medicine.

The Mysterious Power of Parsley. The root of this herb is a prime source of calcium, B-complex vitamins, and iron. These nutrients are released directly into the bloodstream and are sent to nourish the parathyroid glands. These four tiny glands (two on either side of the thyroid) are concerned with regulating the supply of calcium in the body. Parsley herb nutrients go into the endocrine system, nourish the parathyroids, and enter into the making and assimilation of valuable calcium.

In Bertha's situation, parsley root tea helped the parathyroids regulate a steady supply of bone calcium that was "food" for the marrow of the skeletal structure. In this tea was a natural "hormone" that promoted an inner homeostasis (body glandular balance) that eased her arthritic-like stiffness. Nature's medicines had helped promote flexibility and youthfulness of her joints.

PARSLEY TONIC: Pour one quart of boiling water over one cup of firmly packed, fresh parsley, both leaves and stems. Allow to steep 15 minutes. Strain through a coarse sieve. Bottle promptly. Let cool. Refrigerate. Drink just one-half a cup of Parsley Hormone Tonic daily. It reportedly contains natural hormones that stimulate the parathyroids to release their own hormones for overall health and fitness, with a good measure of youthfulness.

How Herbs Nourish Your Glands and Help You
Slim Down Your Figure

A poorly nourished pituitary gland is often found to be responsible for overweight. If this gland is denied its valuable vitamins as well as amino acids, it becomes erratic in its vital functions. It will react through an upset hypothalamus (portion of the pituitary). This hypothalamus, lying directly above the pituitary, reacts by helping to cause irritating behavior in a person as well as appetite derangement or upset. In order to help control a runaway appetite craving satisfaction the hypothalamus needs to be naturally adjusted with hormones and nourishment, to help ease tension and also relax the compulsion to eat.

Henry R. and His Appetite-Control Hormone Tonic. An easily agitated salesman, Henry R., had a compulsion for sweets and snacks. He was so nervous, he would gobble and nibble all day long and in between extra-heavy meals. He gained so much weight, he was soon too fat and was denied additional life insurance. Now he was more nervous than previously. He needed the insurance more now than ever before. But he could not reduce his weight. His problem was a wild appetite. He could not slim down. What to do?

Herbs Soothe the Hypothalamus and Regulate Abnormal Appetite. Henry R. attended the calorie-watching sessions. Group therapy was only of temporary relief. Away from the crowd of "fatties" who were slimming down, he was back to his voracious appetite. But at one such group therapy session, a lecturer told of being able to ease the hypothalamus (labelled the glandular cause of excess weight) by using a special Appetite-Control Hormone Tonic. It was made of all-natural "organic medicines" or just two common but effective herbs—sassafras and burdock.

The root, bark, and seeds of these herbs, when boiled in a tea, release a strong oil that is soothing to the hypothalamus. Furthermore, the ingredients of these two herbs aid the adjacent pituitary gland in releasing an ample supply of protein to help adjust hormone balance in the body.

Henry R. made this Appetite-Control Hormone Tonic as follows: From a local herbal pharmacist or health food store, he obtained a powdered combination of both sassafras and burdock root. He used one-half teaspoon to one cup of boiled water as a tea. He sweetened with a dollop of organic honey. Henry R. would drink this tea throughout the day, eliminating coffee or "commercial" tea.

Herbs Ease Appetite and Help in Slimming Down. The use of this Appetite-Control Hormone Tonic helped calm his much-agitated hypothalamus. Furthermore, it helped send pituitary-like hormones into the body, creating more of an internal homeostasis or body balance. The pituitary, itself, was slowly being "adjusted" to healthy regulation.

Benefits: The soothing relaxation of the "organic hormones" from the herb helped soothe and regulate the pituitary-hypothalamus gland, and, furthermore, it helped ease Henry's appetite. As we note, it was this erratic and uncontrolled hormone misbehavior that had caused a derangement of the pituitary gland action and led to his abnormal craving for sweets. But with the help of the Appetite-Control Hormone Tonic, the gland was healthfully adjusted and his appetite was relaxed and eased.

The Slimming Down Process: His compulsive eating urge was soothed and he could soon slim his weight down. He was able to obtain additional insurance. But—he grew overly confident. He gave up the Appetite-Control Hormone Tonic. Soon, he developed such an obsession for sweets and starches, that he became seriously corpulent. His deranged pituitary-hypothalamus gland again made him emotionally unstable. Now he had to be placed under heavy sedation and chemical therapy, which created undesirable side effects.

Herbal Hormone Tonics

Throughout the centuries, folklore remedies have included herbal hormone tonics as the foundation of youthful health. Today, in the quest for organic medicines, herbs are becoming increasingly popular for their effectiveness in helping the body's glands establish *youthful hormonal rhythm.* Here are a number of time-tested, folklore herbal hormone tonics that reportedly act as "food medicine" for the glands and as nature's hormones for regulating the entire body and mind in turning back the aging clock.

BAYBERRY TONIC. This aromatic shrub possesses mild astringent properties. It is believed to cause a rejuvenation of the adrenal glands, helping to cleanse the bloodstream, wash out age-causing wastes in veins and arteries, and rid the body system of poisonous wastes that rob one's youthfulness.

BITTER ROOT TONIC. While tasting strongly bitter, this herb can be made more palatable with organic honey. It soothes and stimulates the pancreas and improves the sugar-burning process in the body. It helps send a stream of hormones into self-cleansing action, washing out the gall ducts, liver tubuli, and the muscular-mucous membranes of the bowels and kidneys. All parts of the plant contain a milky juice which is often called "Nature's Milk Hormone."

CASCARA SAGRADA TONIC. The Indians called this a "sacred

bark herb." The bark is rich in hormone-like oils which help boost the peristaltic action (pushing out wastes) of the intestinal canal. Through nourishment of the pituitary, it helps this master gland secrete its dozen valuable hormones and maintain internal homeostasis, stepping up the functions of the stomach and liver to youthful activity.

CHAMOMILE TONIC. The whole herb of this healing grass is rich in valuable substances that nourish the glands, especially the thyroid. The benefit here is that the herb helps promote a natural hormone, like that of thyroxine, which helps rejuvenate the texture of hair and skin and also helps boost youthful mental alertness.

WILD CHERRY TONIC. Here is a tasty, fruit-like hormone herb that has special benefits for the thymus. It supplies better nourishment to maintain a healthful calcium-phosphorus balance. Wild Cherry Tonic has organic hormones that help the body manufacture white corpuscles, needed to fight infectious diseases.

CHICKWEED TONIC. In particular, this hormone herb tonic soothes the pineal gland (cone-shaped little organ, suspended by a stalk, just behind the mid-brain), bathing it with a hormone-like oil. This herb tonic offers minerals to the pineal and pituitary gland, helping to promote a youthful appearance and mental outlook.

CLOVER TONIC. Various types of clover are available. This organic grass sends natural hormones to the more distant reaches of the respiratory system. Clover Tonic reportedly eases symptoms of colds, allergies, and bronchial disorders. It helps the body's own glands send forth healing hormones to build resistance to such disorders.

COLTSFOOT TONIC. The flowers, roots, and leaves nourish the endocrines, boost basic health, and send soothing hormones to the cells and tissues.

COMFREY TONIC. Characterized by a sweet and astringent taste, this herb tonic feeds the pituitary; it helps in the calcium-phosphorus balance, promoting strong bones and healthy skin. Because this natural hormone tonic helped strengthen the body skeleton, it was often called "knit bone."

DANDELION TONIC. A rich source of vitamins, it sends healing hormones into the system to help dissolve excessive mucus and sludge. It was once used by herbalists to stimulate a sluggish glandular system to send forth natural hormones to prevent and/or dissolve internal wastes. It is regarded as a good hormone tonic to promote internal cleansing.

FIGWORT TONIC. The leaves, roots, and blossoms of this herb join together to issue hormone-like liquids into the system. This helps soothe the digestive organs. The herbal hormones also cleanse the kidneys. Also known as "scrofula plant," this herb issues a good, hormone-like cleansing fluid throughout the entire body.

GOLDEN SEAL TONIC. Well-known as the "king of hormone tonics," it reportedly boosts the entire endocrine gland network. It sends forth natural hormones to soothe the stomach, bowels, and respiratory organs. Its hormone-like messengers go directly into the bloodstream and help regulate the secreting-excreting functions of the liver. Herbalists have long suggested Golden Seal as a means of boosting a sluggish glandular system and promoting youthful hormonal harmony.

HYSSOP TONIC. The flowering tops and leaves have an essential hormone oil that promotes a generally soothing aperient benefit to the bowels. Hyssop also sends its hormone oils directly into the bloodstream, helping to build resistance to infectious diseases.

JUNIPER TONIC. The oils from this herbal berry help enrich body hormones to soothe the kidneys, bladder, and renal organs. In bygone days, juniper was said to help regulate the endocrine system and help relax bladder unrest. Juniper hormones further serve to ease internal inflammation conditions.

LICORICE TONIC. Select the organic, natural herb of this old and popular hormone herb. The root is rich in hormone-like substances that help boost circulation and stimulate a sluggish glandular network. In particular, licorice acts upon the thyroid gland and helps promote production of thyroxine that is needed to improve body metabolism. The natural ingredients in a licorice tonic help create a natural "hormone supplement," to act as a thyroxine substitute while the glands become better and healthfully adjusted.

Where to Obtain Hormone Herbs

Ask any local health store for desired herbs. Ask any herbalist or herbal pharmacy for organically grown herbs. Look in the classified pages of your local telephone directory under "herbs" for the nearest outlet.

HOW TO MAKE HORMONE HERB TONICS. If at all possible, use natural bottled spring water. Favor water that contains no chlorine-fluorine treatment. Warm a non-metal pot. Pour boiling water over the herb leaves or crushed seed. Steep between five to eight minutes. If a stronger infusion is desired, add more leaves. *Tip:* Use a few leaves of freshly cut herbs or one-half teaspoon of dry crushed herbs for each cup of tonic.

NOTE: If using seeds, then they should be lightly crushed to release their oil-like hormones. Then pour boiling water over the seeds. Let boil from five to 10 minutes.

Sweetening: Organic honey should be used in moderation. You may also want to use a little natural, pure maple syrup to impart a sweet taste to the more pungent types of herbal teas.

The delicate ingredients in herbs help create natural hormone-like supplementation to the endocrine system. Use nature's organic substances as medicines to help improve your health, regain youthfulness, and condition your glands with natural hormones, as no other man-made substance can.

In Review of This Chapter

1. Herbs are nature's own hormones that help supplement the body's glands and promote better health.

2. Slippery elm helps boost the adrenal glands and produces a warming of hands and feet, as well as a youthful skin color, through hormone regeneration. Janet A. found new life with this herbal hormone.

3. Bertha K. was able to activate her pituitary gland with a parsley tonic and relax her "stiff fingers" and "tight joints" with corrective food programs, as well.

4. Hormones in the sassafras and burdock herbs soothed the pituitary-hypothalamus glands, eased the compulsive eating urge for Henry R., and helped him slim down without medicines.

5. Herbal Hormone Tonics are time-tested folklore remedies that reportedly help promote rejuvenation of mind and body through glandular nourishment and natural supplementation.

18

Yoga Secrets for Stimulating Hormones to Promote Youthfulness

As far back as history records, the Hindu mystics have used Yoga to help keep the body and mind as youthful as possible. A newly discovered method of rejuvenation, using the age-old wisdom of the Yoga of the East, says the body needs to be brought into conformity with the laws of nature and then properly adjusted, so it is youthfully responsive to the commands of the mind. Health authorities are beginning to recognize the youth-health benefits of Yoga, and are gradually accepting this mystical program for natural hormone stimulation. The long life and youthful mentality of Yoga practitioners offer hope for a feeling of continuing youthful health through "charging" and "exercising" the endocrine glands, utilizing this ancient secret of Yoga.

How Yoga Helps Stimulate Hormone Production to Restore and Improve Youthful Health

Yoga is the oldest-known health science, originating in the Orient, and was found to be helpful in stimulating hormones that restore and improve youthful health. Yoga is more than a series of exercises and postures. Yoga literally means a "glandular union of mind and body" to help create a feeling of unexcelled physical health and hormone-rejuvenated emotional well-being. The Orientals and Hindus developed some 84 main postures (asanas) or Yoga exercises. The exercises are grouped as either stretching, inversion (head and shoulder stands), balancing, or standing and sitting postures. The Hindus also developed simple breathing exercises and special groupings of other exercises as a means of helping to stimulate the entire endocrine glandular system by restoring a rhythmic flow of youth-building hormones. The overall goal is to boost *hormone harmony*, which will then lead to a youthful feeling.

The Mysterious Hormone Secret of the Hindu Yoga Practitioner

A newly discovered and formerly mysterious secret of the youth-building health of Yoga is that *these simple exercises help the glands reverse the customary pull of gravity on the body's muscles, blood vessels, and lymph glands.* When Yoga exercises help reverse this gravity, glandular benefits as follows are made possible to help stimulate a feeling of youthfulness:

1. *Hormone-Energized Legs.* Yoga exercises help send a flow of youthful hormones to the feet, legs, and thighs. Yoga helps increase the venous flow of blood, boosting the reverse lymph movement *away* from the lower extremities. *Secret Benefit:* This helps speed up the elimination of lactic acid and other by-products of fatigue, creating a feeling of energized legs, thanks to a hormone-washing benefit.

2. *Hormone-Relaxed Muscles.* Yoga exercises relieve the entire body's muscular structure that resists the constant pull of gravity. Yoga exercises further relax the muscles by using hormones to maintain internal balance of the "pull" of gravity. *Secret Benefit:* By helping to maintain musculature homeostasis or balance, hormones bring about a natural relaxation throughout the body.

3. *Hormone Nourishment to Hair and Skin.* Yoga exercises send an increased supply of hormone-carrying blood to the head. This promotes capillary (tiny vein) nourishment of the hair follicles and skin capillaries. *Secret Benefit:* Yoga establishes "balanced gravity" so that hormones can be sent to nourish the most distant reaches of the body. The youthful head of hair and the wrinkle-free health of the skin of most Hindu practitioners of Yoga, who are often close to the 80's, attest to the glandular effectiveness of hormone stimulation for all parts of the body through this ancient health art.

4. *Hormones Boost Youthful Mentality.* The Hindu practices Yoga, knowing that it will send an increased flow of hormone-carry-

ing blood to the brain cells, to bring about their proper aeration and nourishment. This is the secret key to the amazing youthful mentality of many Hindus and Orientals who are Yoga practitioners. *Secret Benefit:* Simple Yoga exercises introduce a stream of fresh oxygen that is absorbed by the bloodstream and blended into the hormones, which then wash and nourish the millions of brain cells. This helps reduce brain fatigue and boosts more youthful mentality for sharper thinking.

In addition to helping restore some youthful body flexibility, the various postures of Yoga work to strengthen and recondition the body through more stimulated hormone functions. Yoga also helps ease tension and gives a healthfully flexible muscle tone through a properly balanced glandular rhythm. The ancient secrets of Yoga are gradually coming into use in our modern daily living and are noted for helping correct many conditions of ill health traced to glandular malfunctioning.

A Simple 10-Minute Yoga Hormone Stimulator for Beginners

The simplest of all Yoga exercises is that of using the *slant board.* Anyone can help boost the health of his body through glandular stimulation, by performing this simple Yoga exercise.

The "Magical" Slant Board. You may purchase a slant board at many health stores. It is a plank that measures about 6 feet long and 18 inches wide. It is slightly padded for your comfort. It is raised at one end to a height of about 15 inches. You may obtain such a slant board at a medical-supply house, pharmacy, or health store.

How to Make Your Own Slant Board. Just obtain a solid board (at any lumberyard or scrap dealer) that is 6 feet long and about 18 inches wide. Merely raise the foot end of this board by placing a low stool or chair directly beneath it. NOTE: It should be raised no higher than 12 to 15 inches.

Simple Rejuvenation Program: Just lie down on this slant board, your head at the lower part, and remain in a comfortable position for as little as 10 minutes or as long as 30 minutes.

How the Slant Board Will Help Stimulate Your Hormones. This simple position reverses the downward hormone pull of the body. It forces the hormones into the more vital centers of the body. When your feet are just 12 to 15 inches higher than your head, the pull of gravity is reversed. Your body hormone fluids are likewise reversed, and are now sent to hitherto inaccessible parts of your body, to promote more youthful nourishment.

Hindu Secret for Youthful Flexibility. The Hindu, as well as many other Oriental practitioners of Yoga, has perfect posture and youthful flexibility at all ages! The slant board exercise, which all Yoga practitioners will perform daily as a starter, helps the spine straighten out and flattens the bent back. Muscles which might be otherwise tense, are now nourished with hormone-impregnated blood, lactic acid is sloughed out, and there is a free feeling of youthful flexibility.

In particular, the slant board exercise frees the feet and legs from their customary burden, and the hormone-induced reverse force of gravity now brings about a release of accumulated congestion in the bloodstream and tissues. This eases the risk of swollen limbs or strained muscles, which predispose to a bent-over, "aging" posture.

By reversing body gravity pull, hormones are now able to reach those formerly inaccessible regions that might otherwise be "starved" and therefore have become prematurely aged. The slant board helps the glands promote this youthful hormone rhythm function.

The Secret of a Secretary's Natural "Face Lift"

Ellen R. looked older than her early 50's. She was one of the first to be given a dismissal as part of a large economy drive in the huge wholesale company where she worked. Ellen R. now found that other companies perferred "youthful looking" secretaries. While she had experience, her appearance made her look unhappily "old," with a sallow and wrinkled skin, drooping features, sagging throat line, and slumped posture. Since appearances are often more important than experience, Ellen R. learned that she was being turned down in favor of younger-looking secretaries who had less training and experience than she had.

How a Natural "Face Lift" Through Hormone Revitalization Was Accomplished. Ellen R. became nervous, required medical treatment, and was told that if she wanted to look younger, she ought to consider plastic surgery. Meanwhile, she was put on a slimming diet (she was also overweight), and this introduced her to more healthful hormone foods as well as an exercise program. She decided she would try to get a natural "face lift" through Yoga. In particular, she followed the elementary 10-minute slant board exercise. Following is how Ellen R. was able to give herself a natural "face lift" with this simple program, based upon the wisdom of ancient Eastern Yoga:

1. Every evening she would spend 15 minutes on her slant board, and then take a refreshing nap.

2. After this easy, "do nothing" exercise (it has an *automatic* hormone gravity action that works while you sleep!), Ellen R. would soak herself in a warm tub of water, scented with bath oil.

3. While in the tub, Ellen R. would practice gradual relaxation of all her limbs and muscles. She would relax her shoulder blades, back, stomach, thighs, calves, and feet. NOTE: It was this relaxation that helped hormones push through hitherto congested areas and send youth-building blood to the clogged (wrinkled) portions of her skin. She would have a tub-relaxation event for about 30 minutes nightly.

4. Afterwards, she would eat healthful foods, prepared as simply and naturally as possible. She would rest an hour after the meal, and then prepare to sleep.

RESULTS: It took some eight weeks of following this daily program until Ellen R. did walk and move with better posture. Her skin was toned up because hormones helped the blood reach the hitherto inaccessible clogged nooks and crannies of her face and throat. Her features perked up youthfully. A flush of healthy hormones made her well-nourished capillaries give her the glow of youth. She not only looked younger, but also she felt younger—and in a big way!

Soon, she was hired as a private secretary by an important executive. True, she could not immediately command a salary as high as some of the younger girls (she finally made it after a little while) but she looked much younger than she did before, thanks to the slant board exercise that sent youth-building hormones to her firmed-up skin. She had used Yoga to help give herself an all-natural "face lift" right at home!

How to Limber Up Your Glands with Yoga

From the mysterious East, we learn that the endocrine glands can be "limbered up" or "exercised" to enable them to send forth an increased supply of youth-stimulating hormones, by following these amazingly simple 12 steps:

1. Fold your hands. Stand tall. Both legs together.

2. Breathe deeply. Lift up your arms. Bend backwards.

3. Breathe out and now bend forward until your hands are touching the floor, directly in line with your feet. Bend over until you are able to touch your knees with your head. You may bend your knees slightly. Don't force yourself. Do the best you can. Lift up again.

4. Breathe deeply. Move your right leg away from your body in a backward pose. Keep your left foot firmly on the floor. Gradually, bend your head to the rear.

5. Breathe deeply and hold your breath. Move your left leg alongside your right. Keep your body in a straight line from head to toe. Gradually exhale.

6. Now, lower yourself to the floor and place both hands flat on the floor. It is a form of Sastanga Namaskar, known as "partial prostration." Slowly place your knees, hands, chest, and forehead on the floor while all else is still in a kneeling pose.

7. Breathe deeply. Bend backwards as comfortably far back as possible.

8. Breathe out. Keep your hands and feet on the floor. Your hips are high. Your heels are flat and your head down.

9. Breathe in deeply. Then breathe out.

10. Breathe in and out. Press down on your hands.

11. Lift your arms over your head. Bend backwards, breathing in.

12. Breathe out, drop your arms, and relax.

BENEFITS: The rhythmic exercises help alert almost all of the body's glands, sending forth a stream of invigorating hormones to various parts of the body. The mystics of the Ancient East knew of the revitalizing values of such exercises and would perform them as a daily ritual. This may well have been the secret of their longevity and youthful appearance, through Yoga-stimulated endocrine glands.

How Alternate Yoga Breathing Sends Oxygen to Your Glands

Next to food, your glands need oxygen in order to send refreshed and properly aerated hormones to all of your body parts. The vigor and youthfulness of your hormones may well be determined by the amount of oxygen available to these internal rivers of flowing youth.

The Yoga mystics were aware of the glandular benefits of oxygen, hence their traditional programs of *pranayama*—the art of "glandular ventilation."

The great Indian mystic, Shivagama, reportedly based his long life and youthful health upon proper *pranayama* exercises, performed for a few moments, each day. This mystic once said, "A more useful science than the science of respiration, a more beneficial science than the science of respiration, a greater friend than the science of respiration *has never been seen nor heard.*"

In just *three* words, Mazda, the supreme god of the Zoro-astrian religion, some 2,500 years ago, emphasized the value of sending oxygen to the glands when he declared, *"Breath is life."*

It was Mazda who reportedly developed the "Alternate Yoga Breathing Exercise" that helped send a stream of life-giving breath and oxygen to the glands. His followers did much to perpetuate this secret of internal rejuvenation. Today, this mystical science has been accepted as a means of helping to promote life-giving oxygen to the glands.

ALTERNATE YOGA BREATHING EXERCISE. This centuries-old self-oxygenation exercise is easily followed in our modern times, right in your own home. Here are the steps:

1. Sit cross-legged on a rug or cushion, on the floor, or in a comfortable chair. Do *not* lean on the back of the chair; let your hands provide whatever support is necessary by resting them in your lap.

2. Breathe in and out through your nose several times slowly. Now take one long, slow breath, followed by a speedy exhalation through your nose. Repeat six times. NOTE: For maximum glandular oxygenation, expel air forcefully with your stomach muscles. This helps recharge your internal organs.

3. With your right hand, place your thumb on your *right* nostril. Keep your third finger ready to press on your *left* nostril.

4. Exhale through your *right* nostril while you use slight pressure to close your *left* nostril.

5. Next inhale through your right nostril, while slight pressure closes your left nostril.

6. Next exhale through your left nostril, followed by inhaling through the left, then exhaling through the right.

Your timing should be comfortably quick but full. NOTE: Take 'twice as long to exhale as to inhale. Repeat the complete cycle three times, making six breaths. Here is your blueprint, as based upon the original Alternate Yoga Breathing Exercise of Mazda, the supreme god of the Zoro-astrians and the reputed "forever youthful" leader of the Indian people:

> out right,
> in right, out left,
> in left, out right,
> in right, out left,
> in left, out right,
> in right, out left,
> in left, out right.

What Mazda's Alternate Yoga Breathing Exercise Will Do to Rejuvenate Your Hormones. The rhythmic breathing sends oxygen, via the hormones, to your body tissues. The oxygenated hormones nourish the hemoglobin of the red blood cells. The oxygenated hormones are then carried through a great vascular network to the microscopic capillaries which permeate the tissues at that point. They diffuse from the blood across the capillary membrane to the tissue, in proportion to the rejuvenating needs of that specific tissue.

Oxygen, as introduced through Mazda's exercise, becomes intimately involved with the biochemical processes which synthesize the primary youthful energy sources. Without sufficient oxygen, those youth-creating processes cannot continue. The tissues become "suffocated" for lack of air and the aging process sets in.

The Mazda breathing exercise helps increase the number and size of the blood vessels that carry the hormones to the body tissue, saturating the tissue throughout your body with youth-building, oxygenated hormones. Do it several times a day, but inhale fresh air only. Do not overdo it; three cycles a day will suffice in most cases.

The Tibetan Yoga Secret for Eternally Young Hormones

From this ancient, mountain-locked land of mystery, comes a secret of special breathing that reportedly gave the holy lamas astonishing youthful health of mind and body, even after they passed the age of 100 years! It is well known that this mystical and occult land possessed secrets of rejuvenation that amazed modern science. Now it has become known that several of their jealously guarded secrets concerned Yoga breathing exercises that would send a powerful supply of rejuvenating oxygen to the glands. Once the glands were properly oxygenated, they could send nourishment to the hormones. The youthful hormones could then help nourish the entire body and promote a feeling of body-mind rejuvenation.

NOTE: The secret of the Tibetan lamas was in being able to build up an "oxygen reserve," just as a food reserve, to be readily available to the hormones. The hormones then worked to improve the body's capacity with sufficient air, delivering it to the tissue cells, where it was combined with foodstuffs to produce youth and vitality. We may well believe that the superior intellect, the mystical genius, and the occult wisdom of the Tibetan lamas and their faithful followers, were traced to properly oxygenated hormones.

SHAVASANA SECRET. Lie flat on your back with feet slightly apart. Relax from head to toe. Place hands on your diaphragm, just below your ribs. *Breathe in* through your nose—slowly, deeply. When your lungs fill slightly, press on your diaphragm to push air into your chest. Fill with air the lower, middle, and upper parts of your lungs. *Breathe out* through your nose—slowly. Gently draw in your stomach at the end of the breathing out. Repeat 10 times.

Benefit of Shavasana Secret. Oxygen becomes combined with energy fuel in the hormone-rejuvenating process known as oxidation. The fuel is now transported to the cells via the hormone stream, where it works to promote overall youthfulness. Oxygen, introduced to the body via the Shavasana Secret, helps stimulate youthful hormones, the key to eternal health, according to the Tibetan lamas.

PURAKA SECRET. The Tibetan word *pūraka* means "filling up" and reportedly will make a "storage supply" of hormone-feeding oxygen in the system. This simple Tibetan exercise is followed in this manner:

Lie flat on your back. Breathe steadily up to five times.

Now breathe out strongly, followed by *breathing in*, using small vigorous sniffs until the lungs are full.

Repeat three times.

Benefit of Puraka Secret. This simple Tibetan exercise makes more oxygen available to the hormones, which work to improve cardiac response, help send "air" to the muscles, and facilitate the removal of waste products, particularly the age-causing carbon dioxide gas in the body. The *Pūraka Secret* creates a "storage bank" of oxygen to help meet the demands of daily living and help the glands maintain a rhythmic amount of youth-building hormones. This Tibetan exercise rightfully offers a "filling up" of oxygen-carrying hormones.

SHAUCHA SECRET. The Tibetan word *shaucha* means "cleanliness." The lamas were well aware of the youth-building benefits of cleaning out the glands and hormones through Yoga exercises. Here is how they would perform the Shaucha Secret amongst themselves and a chosen few:

Sit cross-legged. Breathe normally. Make a "big belly" to bring down or lower your diaphragm. Inhale about a third of a lungful of air.

Forcefully pull in your stomach; at the same time *forcefully* expel all the air in your lungs through your nose.

Quickly take another partial breath through your nose, while you force out your "big belly" again.

When your stomach cannot protrude further, speedily and *forcefully* expel air through your nose, and with simultaneous forcefulness, pull your stomach in.

NOTE: You should establish a steady rhythm to help properly "cleanse" or "wash" your glands. The emphasis is upon the *forceful* expulsion of air through your nose and the simultaneous, vigorous sucking in of your stomach muscles. It is this steady rhythm that the Tibetan lamas regarded as a mystical "cleansing" that washed and stimulated the glands and made them feel youthfully fresh. *TIP:* The Tibetan lamas would perform the *Shaucha Secret* in the morning before breakfast to cleanse the internal organs for accomplishing the day's demands more effectually.

Benefit of Shaucha Secret: This self-cleansing Yoga exercise actually scrubs away phlegm, residues, and impurities, washes them loose from the respiratory system, and enables them to be cast out. The Yoga exercise also "massages" the glands clean so they can work more efficiently to produce more vigorous hormones of youthfulness.

The "Yoga Break" That Makes a Businessman Think Young for Greater Success

Twice daily, Roger T., a much-pressured businessman, takes a "Yoga Break" that sends a stream of oxygen-carrying hormones throughout his nerve and tissue cells, giving him a "think young" stimulus. Here are the exercises as Roger T. does them, right in the privacy of his own office or the company rest lounge:

1. *Nerve-Strengthener.* Stand, legs apart. Inhale slowly. Exhale—

and while exhaling, raise both arms forward to shoulder height, with palms turned upwards. Close hands into fists. Hold breath. Pull clenched hands strongly back to shoulder height. Repeat five times. *Benefit:* Roger T. stretches out his arms as if held back by an invisible opposing power, to help boost effectiveness. This Yoga exercise sends oxygen-rich hormones to soothe the nervous system and helps control "jittery fingers" and nervous trembling.

2. *Mental Rejuvenation.* Stand, legs apart. Take a full breath while you slowly lift your arms above your head. Hold your breath for the count of five. Now, quickly bend forward at the waist. Relax your arms. Let them drop loosely. Now exhale strongly through your *mouth,* forming the sound "Ha." *Next,* breathe slowly through your nose, lift up, raise arms above head, and then breathe out through your *nose*—afterwards, drop your arms. *Benefit:* Roger T. feels a speeded up hormonal-blood circulation and a stimulation of the respiratory organs. This is especially beneficial as it "ventilates" the glands and helps provide oxygen to indoor workers. It also helps boost the mental faculties for keen thinking.

3. *Brain Invigoration.* Sit or stand. (This may be done right at your desk.) The tip of your tongue touches the upper palate. Breathe in through your mouth with a hissing sound. Hold your breath for the count of five. Then breathe out slowly through the nose. *Benefit:* Repeat regularly, whenever you feel a "tightness" or "brain fatigue." The oxygen goes speedily into the glands and the hormones, which go hurrying to the brain to send "air" and invigoration. Roger T. maintains that this Brain Invigoration is almost as good as taking a walk in the open air! It's refreshing and it helps him "bounce back" with "think young" hormones.

While Roger T. is able to lick executive stress and is able to improve his thinking facilities with Yoga, he only follows the glandular rejuvenation in a limited form. He scoffs at natural health laws, he shrugs off natural foods, he uses only the Yoga segment of health restoration through hormone nourishment. As a consequence, Roger T. enjoys a partial feeling of youthfulness. He is beset with fears that his younger competitors will take away his job. He has become jealous of their successes. His unhealthy attitudes, together with unhealthy food-living habits, are undermining his strength. Yoga exercises offer some help, but they need the back-up power of *all* the natural laws of hormonal living.

Secrets of the Yoga Sages: The mystical wise men of the Middle

East and the Far East have long recognized that the quality of the hormones (although they may not have identified these youth substances by this modern name) depends largely on the quantity of oxygen absorbed by the lungs. The Yoga sages hold that improper breathing will impede the quantity and quality of hormone production. This will also affect the body organisms. In particular, the digestive organs need hormone-carrying oxygen for proper functioning. Denied oxygen in this form, the digestive system malfunctions and poor absorption of nutrients leads to premature aging. The hormones, hold the mystical Tibetan lamas and the wise Yoga leaders, must ge given rhythmical supplies of oxygen, as set out in this chapter.

Unique Secret: The Yoga teachers felt that breathing is an alternation between a positive-negative state in the hormones. Namely, *breathing out* is a positive state during which the hormones take energy to be distributed to most body parts. *Breathing in* is a negative state in which the hormones are receptive and waiting for proper oxygen.

Yoga mystical leaders knew that the secret of youthful health lay in being able to regulate consciously the uniformity of the breathing process. They called for establishing a *balance* between the positive and negative vibrations. The principal variations, as revealed in the different exercises in this chapter, are said to provide the "breath of life" to the glands and help promote youthful hormones.

In the words of Sivananda, the great Yoga mystic, "Yoga insures beauty, health, strength, and long life."

Highlights

1. Mystical Yoga practitioners maintained that simple exercises had four special youth-building benefits through hormone stimulation.

2. A simple 10-minute Yoga exercise can help improve the rhythm of your hormone rivers.

3. Ellen R. underwent a natural "face lift" through a unique four-step hormone stimulation program.

4. Just 12 simple, time-tested steps, drawn from ancient archives, help limber up the body glands through Yoga.

5. Alternate Yoga breathing, as practiced in Tibetan monasteries, helps send youth-giving oxygen to the glands, promoting better body-mind health.

6. Mazda's Yoga secret is now available for your home use.

7. The Tibetan Yoga Secret is the legendary mystery for "eternally young" hormones. Try it at home, a few moments each day.

8. The three gland-breathing programs, Shavasana Secret, Pūraka Secret, Shaucha Secret, drawn from Tibetan scrolls, reportedly wash-rejuvenate the glands and boost the flow of youthfully clean hormones.

9. A "Yoga Break" may help give you youthful energy, as it does for Roger T.

19

How to Self-Massage Your Glands for a Youthful Flow of Energizing Hormones

S elf-massage is a gland-stimulating method that has been known as far back as Classical Greece, and perhaps even earlier. Self-massage helps to stimulate the glands, promoting a more rhythmic flow of youthful hormones. By means of comfortably deep finger and hand pressures on accessible body parts, self-massage invigorates the hormones to help remove excess wastes that have collected because of sluggish glandular function. Self-massage helps the circulation of hormones in the areas of congestion. Once a fresh supply of blood-carrying hormones are brought into "tight pockets" of congestion, there is a youthful circulation that helps send nutritive, rebuilding materials to the tissues. The liberated hormones are able to promote the removal of excess fluids and tissue debris that may be part of the premature aging process.

Self-massage has a unique benefit, in that it aids in the breakdown of age-causing adhesions. The hormones are then able to "swim" into the "choked" region and help remove these adhesions through absorption. If there is a sluggish hormone condition, these non-elastic adhesions will remain and interfere with the elasticity of the surrounding tissues. Prolonged hormone deprivation may lead to an accumulation of such age-causing adhesions until they choke off free-flowing circulation. Ill health may then be the consequence. Small wonder that the ancients placed such value on self-massage as a means of helping to prolong the look and feel of youth. The hormone flow induced did the work.

10 Gland-Awakening Benefits of Self-Massage

While the overall body-mind benefits of hormonal stimulation through self-massage are usually felt rather quickly, the more lasting gland-awakening benefits occur after continued practice. There are, however, 10 special gland-awakening benefits of self-massage, that should make this ancient health therapy a valuable part of your natural program. These 10 benefits are:

1. Self-massage sends hormones to your voluntary muscular system, helping to give the muscles more elasticity and ease tension spots. The hormones help to soothe tight muscle spasms.

2. Perked-up glands send hormones to those body parts that help increase the number of red blood cells. In particular, the hemoglobin in the bloodstream becomes enriched when sufficient hormones are available as nourishment. It is self-massage that helps send a fresh stream of valuable blood-building hormones to most body regions.

3. Sluggish blood circulation becomes youthfully increased by activation of "sleepy" glands through self-massage. In particular, self-massage along the veins helps in the dilatation (opening) of the capillaries to promote a more youthful blood circulation.

4. Self-massage invigorates the balanced rhythm of lymph. The lymphatic system runs in an approximate parallel to that of the blood vessels, becoming connected in the upper chest. Self-massage helps the glands send lymph flowing in all valuable directions, through the body's valves and nodes and in the lymphatic tubular system. Self-massage helps to direct the lymph into its own channels (it may otherwise stray from the lymph tubes and invade surrounding tissues possibly promoting serious health combinations), and also helps to increase its vigor. The hormones act as "batteries" to regulate this internal rhythm of keeping the healthy youth-promoting lymph in its own lymphatic vessels and maintain body homeostasis (balance).

5. A unique benefit of self-massage is that the steady stroking or kneading helps raise skin temperature and soothe the nervous system. In particular, the hormones work to expand the skin capillaries, then to nourish the superficial tissues. This helps rejuvenate the appearance, complexion, and texture of the skin and scalp.

6. Gentle self-massage strokes help soothe peripheral nerves. (The nerves at the outside end or periphery of the total nervous system.) This enables the stimulated hormones to soothe the *nerve ends.* Self-massage gives these nerve ends a "tingling" feeling that is overall relaxing and soothing.

7. Self-massage sends hormones to the central nervous system to help promote an internal balance that offers a *natural sedative* to relax tense body parts. Often, it may even help induce healing sleep.

8. Self-massage sends "hormone cleansers" to float away the toxic by-products of muscular exertion. Once hormones wash away these lactic acid by-products, there is a gradual relaxation of nervous tension.

9. Elimination becomes more regular through self-massage. An adjusted glandular network will help in sending off excess nitrogen and sodium chloride that may cause internal tissue destruction. The glands send their hormones to help wash away these nitrogenous substances, along with irritating excesses of sodium chloride (salt), easing internal tensions.

10. General self-massage alerts the glands to help create better oxygen consumption. The hormones transport youth-giving oxygen to the lungs, the brain, and the other vital organs. Once these organs receive valuable "breathing" nourishment via the hormones, they are able to function more efficiently.

CAUTION: Under certain conditions, self-massage should not be used. These include problems of swelling, acute inflammation, skin eruptions, varicose veins, pain, pregnancy, and prolonged bed-ridden confinement. For any conditions of ill health, self-massage should be followed *only* with your doctor's personal approval and advice.

Four Easy Ways to Tune Up Your Glands with Self-Massage

To help tune up your glands with self-massage, here are the four most recognized ways in which you can stimulate your hormones and help improve a youthful feeling of body and mind:

1. STROKING. Use long, firm, rhythmic strokes on any accessible body parts. Cup the palm of your hand and fingers. Make light pressure as you stroke **toward** your heart, in the direction of the veins' circulation. Your pressure should be uniform. Stroke in the direction of a muscle, but never across it.

2. KNEADING. This is a manipulation of the muscles. You grasp, roll, squeeze, press, and lift accessible muscles between the palms of both hands. Or, squeeze between the thumb and fingers of one hand. Use gentle and rhythmic pressures. *Always* work in a direction toward the head. Your kneading tempo should be that of stroking broadly.

3. FRICTION. Place your flat palms over skin surfaces. Move your skin and surface tissues over the bone or the deeper structures. Use rotary movements. After five completed circles, move your palms to an adjacent region without lifting from the skin. Keep up these rotary-circular movements. NOTE: Use firm palm pressure that will move your tissues but do *not* bruise yourself. Maintain a broad, ·stroking, steady rhythm.

4. PERCUSSION. You cup your hands and beat lightly against your skin. This self-massage technique consists of light blows delivered alternately by each hand. Move up and down and continue only until the skin develops a slight coloration.

SUGGESTION: Here are four variations of *Percussion:*

A. *Hacking.* Strike your muscle fibres briskly with the little-finger edge of each hand in turn.

B. *Pounding.* With a half-closed fist, strike your various body parts.

C. *Tapping.* With extended fingertips, tap sharply on the skin surfaces in a peck-peck-peck rhythm.

D. *Slapping.* Use cupped palm and fingers and "punctuate" your skin surfaces.

SELF-MASSAGE IS PREFERRED. When you self-massage, you are able to determine any degree of discomfort and can adjust the force of the pressure. This helps ease the threat of hurt or pain. Take care not to injure your capillaries or otherwise bruise delicate tissues. Many a tender-skinned person can emerge with black-and-blue marks from an over-ambitious masseur, so if you do your own massaging, be careful and gentle to help improve your physiological processes.

Self-massage helps tune up your glands in the previously described four easy ways and may be followed just a few moments each day, in conjunction with the other described programs, to help your body adjust its biological gland clocks and promote youthful hormones.

A QUICK "PICK-ME-UP" MASSAGE. Roy P. is under extreme tension as a multiple-duties executive for a large trucking company. After a difficult day at the office or factory, he finds relief from this simple self-massage program that takes *only five minutes* of time:

He makes 10 "stroking" motions across his forehead in both directions. He uses his fingertips. He follows this with stronger full-finger stroking from the back of his neck to the top of his head. He usually does 10 motions of each of these self-massage exercises. Roy P. finishes with firm kneading of the muscle at the juncture of the neck and each shoulder.

Benefit: He unlocks the taut arterial-neuron intersections, and helps send a stream of relaxing hormones that ease tension and give him a natural "pick-me-up" feeling.

HOW SELF-MASSAGE HELPS ESTABLISH REGULARITY. Problems of constipation are often traced to congestion of the colonic region in the pelvic area. While constipation should be relieved by corrective food programs that include fibrous green vegetables, dry bulk foods, and fresh, raw fruit, it will also respond to glandular "regularity."

Self-massage helps use the glands to alert the drawstring-like muscles that close the rectum of the anus. Hormones work to activate the sympathetic nervous system, to relax any nervous spasms or rigidity that may be part of the constipation problem.

Simple, Easy Self-Massage. Press fingertips of both hands into your abdomen, working toward the right side, near the appendix. Knead the muscles with a circular movement some five times. Dig deeper on your upstroke. Be gentle on your downstroke. Continue the circular motions upwards until you reach your rib line. Now make the rotary motions to your left, with slightly more gentle pressure on the leftward strokes than on the return.

When you reach the far left of your stomach, move downward with the steady circular kneading, until you reach your hip joint. Here, stop your circular motions.

With your right-hand fingers, make a deep slanting stroke to a position 4 inches below your navel. Repeat the same slanting 10 times.

In all, this should take about *two minutes.* This self-massage alerts the sluggish hormones in the pelvic region to flow through the locked channels and helps promote natural regularity. In particular, the glands work to "hormonize" the tight drawstring-like muscles that are too constricted and prohibit natural bowel movements. Once these muscles are relaxed by hormones that are stimulated through self-massage, a pattern of regularity may be established. This Simple-Easy Self-Massage for Regularity of Bowel Movement may be performed in the morning, before breakfast.

HOW SELF-MASSAGE EASES HEADACHES. Myrna B., an overly active clubwoman housewife, den mother, and part-time bookkeeper, is frequently beset with tension headaches. Rather than take aspirins, which she finds upsetting to her digestion, she follows this program:

Headache-Eze Self-Massage: Press fingertips of both hands against the forehead at the hairline. Move in small circles—the right hand is clockwise, the left hand is counter-clockwise. The skin and muscles move until the frontal bone can be felt. Repeat for the count of 10. Next, move spread fingertips higher and repeat. Continue until the op of the head is reached. Now drop down behind your ears and repeat the same circular motions. When you reach the mastoid bump, go downward. Repeat for a total of five minutes.

Myrna B. claims that this helps ease problems of pounding headaches and the nerve-wracking tension of a stiff neck that follows at the end of a hard day's work.

FAVORITE FOOT MASSAGE. To be your own masseur and bring relief to tired feet, here's what you do. Sit down. Cross your ight leg over your left knee. Use both hands. Knead your toes. Take each toe, one at a time, and knead from the tip to the juncture with the sole. Next, clasp your right foot with both hands. Your fingers should meet above the instep. Your thumbs should be together under the sole. Stroke firmly from your toes toward your heel. Unclasp your hands at each stroke end as you return to the starting point. Maintain a rhythmic motion.

Next, clasp your right foot just beneath the ankle with the thumb and fingers of your left hand astride the Achilles tendon; your right hand presses on your instep. Stroke firmly upward to the beginning of your calf. Repeat up to 12 times.

Uncross your legs and relax for a few moments.

Next, cross your left leg over your right knee and repeat the same self-massage process, but with your left foot.

Benefit: This Favorite Foot Massage helps the glands send a supply of hormones through the veins that siphon off the by-products of tiredness. The hormones invigorate the circulatory networks and refresh the miles of blood and lymph vessels, helping to melt tired legs and promote a youthful resiliency to your feet.

HOW TO SELF-MASSAGE AWAY LEG CRAMPS. Jayne E. is troubled with muscular seizures called cramps. Here's her technique to help self-massage away leg cramps:

Immerse both legs in a warm (not hot) tub, with the water coming up to the knees. Keep knees slightly bent. With both hands, knead the leg muscles, beginning below the painful area and working up toward the knee. Fingers should connect at the shinbone, while both thumbs alternately provide deep pressure against the calf as they climb higher. There should be a rhythmic series of kneading and stroking upward with the palms of both hands. With the leg weight resting on the heel, work up and down your foot about 12 times Repeat with second foot.

Benefit: Leg cramps may often arise from imperfect hormonal drainage of fatigue by-products that have become clogged in the lower limbs. When immersed in water, self-massage helps the legs achieve "internal gravity." The massage liberates hormones into the bloodstream, to pour into the clogged regions and help ease the spasmodic contractions of tight muscles and leg cramps.

Jayne E. finds welcome relief by following this self-massage for leg cramps technique. The difficulty here is that she must stand for hours and hours on her working job. This leads to increasing congestion and recurring pains. However, Jayne E. is grateful for partial relief through this all-natural method.

VENUS BOSOM MASSAGE. Legend has it that the beauteous Venus, goddess of love, used self-massage in order to help firm up her bosom. Whether or not it was true, we do know that she served as the inspiration for thousands of Greek women who would use self-massage to help lift up and strengthen the supporting pectoral muscles. The benefit here is that self-massage alerts a sluggish hormonal flow. The health of the glands and hormones attest to firm breasts in the female. Self-massage is "exercise" for these glands.

Breast-Support Muscle Massage. Both hands begin at the sternum (breastbone). Lightly stroke the pectoral muscles as they move diagonally toward the shoulder joints. Increase the stroking pressure as you round the top of the shoulders and work to meet at the upper spine. As your hands return, stroke firmly over the shoulders, drawing the muscles toward the front of the neck. Lighten finger-stroking pressure as you come back to the breastbone.

SUGGESTION: Many professional masseurs will make circles with their fingertips as they move their hands in progression from the breastbone to the shoulders in six circles. The right hand moves clockwise. The left hand moves counter-clockwise. Vary the pressure so it is light as the fingers are on the upper portion, but slightly heavier as they reach downward.

Many flat-chested women hope to develop more attractive contours through injected-estrogen therapy. While hormone injections may bring about some beneficial results, there are risks of side effects. The body's hormone balance is set up in so hair-trigger a fashion that unwise synthetic injections may cause internal upheaval. Many doctors agree that stimulation of the body's natural hormones through self-massage, corrective food programs, and better living methods, are much more in keeping with helping the body aid in its own glandular manufacture. For those flat-chested women who seek a Venus bosom, it is best to seek "natural estrogen therapy" through natural foods, natural living methods, and self-massage, as outlined in this book.

Important Benefits from This Chapter

1. Self-massage is an ancient gland-stimulating method that helps improve the rhythmic flow of natural hormones.

2. Ten gland-awakening benefits of self-massage help promote youthful hormones from head to toe.

3. How to tune up your glands with four easy self-massage techniques.

4. The Quick "Pick-Me-Up" Massage that helps restore youthful vitality to a tired head and "knotty" neck.

5. Self-massage may help establish freedom from constipation by unlocking tight rectal-anal muscles.

6. The Headache-Eze Self-Massage helps relax Myrna B.'s pounding head.

7. Favorite Foot Massage helps promote youthful resiliency in the feet.

8. Jayne E. self-massages away leg cramps with a simple home program.

9. The ancient Venus Bosom Massage may be nature's secret for a lovely bust through natural estrogen via massage.

20

A Summary Home Guide to Natural Hormone Foods for a Full Measure of Youthful Health

A recent discovery in science reveals that the glandular clock action can be healthfully controlled by a unique, all-natural method known as Circadian Rhythm. Natural living programs help create a balanced Circadian Rhythm that promotes youthful hormones. This Rhythm is a built-in body clock that regulates your daily life cycle. When this body clock is out of tune, then the Circadian Rhythm is upset and the hormone output is consequently maladjusted. The key to youthful hormones would be a healthful regulation of this body clock or gland regulation.

Glandular Rhythm Can Be Established by Natural Programs. Your body, including your brain, is ruled by the glandular clocks. Natural health programs help adjust these clocks to perform in a youthful manner. Modern scientists call this glandular rhythm the Circadian Rhythm—from the Latin *circa* (about) and *dia* (day)—or about a day. The natural programs are able to help establish glandular rhythm to promote youthful health throughout the day. These same programs help set up a *regulated* or *measured* hormone movement that offers a look and feel of sustained youthfulness throughout the day. The Circadian Rhythm requires more healthful rules for everyday living, rather than just an occasional program that offers only partial benefits. You will derive more youthful health by fitting these natural health programs into your plans for daily living.

Help your glandular clocks tick forth a steady 24-hour rhythm of youthful hormones with a pattern of natural health programs. Here are some reminders for you in summary form. Please refer to the index for more particular usages.

Golden Dozen Miracle Hormone Foods

GRAPES. A healthful supply of natural fruit sugar together with soothing bioflavonoids and vitamins join with minerals and enzymes to furnish energy fuel to the glands, enabling them to send forth youthful hormones. Grapes and fresh grape juice should be part of the natural health program to promote healthful hormones.

BEANS, PEAS. In particular, obtain the garbanzo or chick-pea bean. Here is a natural food that is rich in magnesium to help the hormones correct excess acidity in the bloodstream. The hormones use the minerals in the garbanzo to strengthen the bones, to assimilate phosphorus, to nourish the respiratory tract. In particular, the hormones need the alkaline content of garbanzos to help establish a healthful acid-alkaline balance. *Cooking Procedure:* To prepare, soak garbanzos or chick-peas in cold water overnight. Next morning, steam at low heat until soft. Add seasonal vegetables or herbs, steam a few moments, then eat as a healthful, mineral-vitamin-protein-rich food for the glands.

ROSE HIPS. From the forests and mountains of Scandinavia, the fruit of the rose plant (a tiny golden-colored fruit) is available in the form of rose hips. Health stores sell rose hips in powder or tablet form. Rich in protein, vitamins (especially Vitamin C), and minerals, they offer a peculiar but potent source of nourishment to the tissues and cells of the body's glands. Citric and malic acids are then taken up by the hormones to promote a youthful glow in the skin. Rose hips may be used in the form of tea (available in tea bags) or as a natural sweetener as a healthful sugar substitute. Perhaps the forever youthful skin glow of Scandinavians may be attributed to their intake of rose hips.

HERBS. These are nature's own hormone medicines, also known as "green magic" because of their unusual healing powers. Of late, modern science has tapped the wisdom of the fields and forests and has used herbs for medications. Herbs are "medicines" for the glands, giving them vital substances which enter into the youthful power of the glands. From any herbal pharmacy, obtain herbs for use as seasonings, spices, or for teas. Use herbs singularly or in combination.

SESAME SEEDS. This remarkable gland food from the Orient and Middle East is a rich source of non-acid proteins, minerals, and especially of the youth-building Vitamin E. NOTE: Sesame seed protein is an alkaline type in contrast to acid-forming protein. The glands need this alkaline protein from sesame seeds for helping to regulate the Circadian Rhythm in a smooth balance. Try sesame seeds in baking; hulled sesame seeds may be munched raw, sprinkled on salads, cereals, soups, or used in sandwiches. Truly a potent gland food!

SEED SPROUTS. The Oriental secret of "eternal youth" and fertility in advanced years may well be in these homemade seed sprouts. The substances in the sprouts are glandularly metabolized and find their way into the hormones, themselves. This may well be the secret of Oriental youth at all ages. Sprouted seeds should be eaten daily as part of the natural health programs for young glands.

APPLE CIDER VINEGAR. The apple has long been hailed as a source of youthful vitality. Apples and their freshly prepared apple cider vinegar is a healthful source of vitamins and minerals. These substances are used by the hormones to promote an antiseptic action to cleanse the digestive tract. The hormones use the apple cider vinegar substances for helping to boost digestion, improve better metabolism, enrich the bloodstream, and strengthen the cells and tissues of the skin. SUGGESTION: For a healthful Hormone Tonic, take one teaspoon of apple cider vinegar in a glass of bottled spring water. Add two tablespoons of honey. Stir vigorously. Drink one hour *before* meals. This enables your digestive glands to "clean sweep" the insides and prepare your stomach for the assimilation process that is to occur. Actually, apple cider vinegar in this Hormone Tonic may well be *a miracle digestive aid from nature.*

CAROB MEAL. The carob tree has been known for thousands of years. Legend has it that the people of the Bible would often subsist entirely upon the carob fruit during their long and arduous journies. Today, we know that the carob fruit is a rich source of natural food, has a quickly assimilable alkaline substance, and contains a treasure of vitamins and minerals. Your hormones welcome this balanced natural hormone food for healthful energizing. Carob is available at health stores in the form of powder. Use it as a sugar substitute. It tastes and even resembles chocolate. It is very delicious in a milk shake. Or, use carob in baking bread, rolls, cookies, waffles, and puddings.

SUNFLOWER SEED. A remarkable plant that is *heliotropic,* or turns toward the sun from dawn till late at night. This process enriches the sunflower plant so that its seeds are regarded as the most potent source of health for the glands. In particular, the sunflower seeds are nature-protected by a hard skin so they resist germs and sprays. The sunflower seeds may be munched raw, ground up as meal for baking, sprouted, or sprinkled over baked goods. Sunflower seeds offer the glands a sun-drenched source of nutrients that may make this wonder food the almost perfect gland energizer.

HONEY. A readily assimilated form of sugar, natural, organic honey is rich in many vitamins, minerals, and some amino acids. Honey is gently soothing to the glands. It acts as a revitalizer by helping the glands send forth a steady and rhythmic supply of youth-building hormones. Honey has long been hailed as a highly beneficial food for the glands and the basic source of youthful energy. Use honey in place of sugar and your glands will reward you with youthful hormones.

MILLET. Here is a whole grain that is an all-around, life-sustaining hormone food with an alkaline reaction. In contrast to other grains, which are acid-forming, this millet grain helps maintain internal balance. Use it as a porridge for breakfast, or as a meal in itself. Obtain organic millet, boil in water until the water has evaporated, then eat the soft millet with a little honey to taste. Millet as a morning grain helps stimulate your glands to send forth healthful hormones for most of the day.

FRESH JUICES. Fresh fruit and vegetable juices supply substances to your glands without the need of expending the same degree of energy on the digestive system that complicated foods require. Juices give your glands a speedy "pickup" and send forth a healthful supply of invigorated hormones to establish a youthful Circadian Rhythm of body and mind. Daily, drink several glasses of freshly prepared fruit or vegetable juices. Your glands will be grateful!

The Golden Dozen Miracle Hormone Foods should be used in your program for helping to improve the health and vitality of your endocrine glands. By allying yourself with nature, your glands will respond to the youth-building Circadian Rhythm.

Hormone Hydrotherapy at Home

Over 20 centuries ago, the highly regarded Roman physician, Asclepiades, observed that youthful health is often obtained through healthful bathing. His knowledge is part of today's medical discovery that hydrotherapy at home can, indeed, promote youthful health through glandular activation and hormone manufacture. Here are ways in which you can bathe your way to youthful hormones through hydrotherapy at home:

Oil Bath. Just a handful of any seed oil (olive, wheat germ, peanut, corn, sunflower) in a tub of water is soothingly relaxing to your glands and skin. Immerse yourself in an Oil Bath for just 30 minutes nightly, and your glands will enjoy a feeling of euphoria which enables them to send forth a rhythmic supply of youthful hormones.

Sulphur Bath at Home. Obtain "flowers of sulphur" from any herbal pharmacist. Gather up one handful and toss into a tub of water that is slightly above body temperature, or from 101°F. to 103°F. Soak yourself up to 15 minutes in this homemade Sulphur Bath. Then, add some cool water to lower the temperature to 94°F. or thereabouts. Rest some 10 minutes. Then let the water run out while you're still in the tub. *Benefit:* The skin pores admit a supply of soothing minerals that are stimulating to the glands and enable them to send forth healthful and youth-building hormones.

Sea Bath at Home. Salt water therapy for glandular revitalization is a widely accepted medical prescription. If you're unable to go to the seashore, try this homemade Sea Bath. At any herbal pharmacist, ask for a natural brine bath powder—or Epsom salt, or just pour in common table salt in a tub of warm water. TIP: Obtain *sea salt* from a health store and enjoy a pseudo-ocean bath right in your own tub! The glands delight in this natural therapy of mineral-rich sea salt.

Epsom Baths. Ordinary Epsom salt is especially beneficial to the glands. Actually, Epsom salt consists of a magnesium sulphate molecule connected to seven water molecules. These water molecules dissolve and give the magnesium sulphate a healing quality. These substances are absorbed by the skin and serve to stimulate he peripheral nerve endings of the glands and capillaries. The glands then send forth a unique type of hormones that have a youthful effect on the body. The end result is a feeling of youthful vitality. To ake an Epsom Bath at home, just pour about two cups of Epsom salt into the tub while the lukewarm water is pouring. Fill the ub. Then immerse yourself and relax up to 15 minutes. Let water run out. Sponge off with free-flowing, comfortably cool water.

You will be delighted at the feeling of youthful imulation mad available to tired muscles and worn-out erves by simple hormone hydrotherapy at home. It was a favorite "revitalizer" of the ancient Greeks and Romans and is today's more popular means of rejuvenation through nature.

The Controlled Fasting Way to Natural Hormones

Controlled fasting is an ancient and time-tested healing program that enables the digestive processes to rest, thereby helping the biological glands establish a soothing Circadian Rhythm. To benefit from fasting, devote just one day to fresh fruits—in the form of juices or as a salad. Just fruits alone for one day will help nourish the body, promote internal cleansing, and help regulate the time-precision functions of the glands.

On another day, have a fresh vegetable fast—drink vegetable juices and eat fresh vegetables throughout the day. This helps the glands metabolize the substances in vegetables *without* interference or "competition" from other foods, thereby helping to boost their assimilation. Just one day on either a fruit or vegetable fast will do much to help boost hormone harmony.

Hormone Harmony While You Sleep

When you enjoy a healthful night of sleep, your glands are able to enjoy rest and relaxation from frenetic daytime pressures. Your glands react to the tensions of the day just as do your nerves and emotions. Sleep is essential for your glands, since they are able to rest up and reward you with more refreshing vigor the next day.

To enjoy better sleep, try to take a short nap during the day to take off the sharp edge of irritation. A daily nap is most beneficial and will actually help you sleep better at night.

Your mattress should not be too soft, as this may cause muscular sagging and spinal curvature. When the body suffers from misalignment, the glands are unable to work efficiently and the result is less-than-perfect hormones. SUGGESTION: You might insert a sleeping board beneath your mattress. Also, you might eliminate a pillow. Sleeping on a high pillow strains your neck and causes spinal curvature and misalignment of the body glands. High pillows further lessen the flow of blood to the head, impeding natural health. You'll sleep better on a thin, soft pillow—or no pillow at all.

Avoid heavy meals just before retiring. The glands must work in the process of assimilation and will keep you tossing and turning until their tasks are done. Instead, take your final meal of the day (make it a light one) some five hours before retiring.

The last few hours of the day should be devoted to peace and quiet. Relax with some soft music, a gentle book, a peaceful walk. In order to enjoy physical and mental harmony with your glands, treat them gently and soothingly and enjoy a healthful night of sleep. You'll be rewarded when you awaken with a refreshed feeling in the morning when your glands are properly tuned up with youthful hormone rhythm.

Natural hormones do hold the secret of youthful health. The purpose of allying with nature is to help the glands promote the highest possible state of youthful health. This calls for nourishing the physical, mental, and emotional components of the body, since all are vitally influenced by the youth and health of the glands. *Indeed, you are as young as your glands.* Feed and ventilate them properly, and you will then be rewarded with a feeling of youthful health of body and mind as long as the glands are youthful. While nutrition is not the sole factor in helping your glands achieve youthful health, without nutrition it is well nigh impossible. So it is with the other described laws of healthful living, which include proper exercise, massage, hydrotherapy, and corrective hormone food programs. When followed fully, they offer hope for sustained youthfulness through natural hormones, as programmed for you in this book.

Index